Workbook

Essentials of Dental Assisting

Fourth Edition

Debbie S. Robinson, CDA, MS
Visiting Research Scholar
Department of Operative Dentistry
School of Dentistry
University of North Carolina
Chapel Hill, North Carolina

Doni L. Bird, CDA, RDH, MA
Director of Allied Dental Education
Santa Rosa Junior College
Santa Rosa, California

D0556598

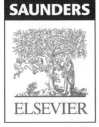

SAUNDERS

ELSEVIER

SAUNDERS
ELSEVIER

11830 Westline Industrial Drive
St. Louis, Missouri 63146

WORKBOOK FOR ESSENTIALS OF DENTAL ASSISTING

ISBN-13: 978-1-4160-4041-5
ISBN-10: 1-4160-4041-2

Notice

ISBN-13: 978-1-4160-4041-5
ISBN-10: 1-4160-4041-2

Senior Editor: John Dolan
Managing Editor: Jaime Pendill
Publishing Services Manager: Pat Joiner
Senior Project Manager: Rachel E. Dowell
Design Direction: Amy Buxton
Cover Designer: Ron Leighton/Bill Smith Studio

Printed in the United States of America

Last digit is the print number: 9 8 7 6 5 4 3 2 1

Contents

Introduction

This student workbook is designed to help you prepare for and master the preclinical, clinical, and administrative procedures presented in *Essentials of Dental Assisting*, Fourth Edition. It is designed so the pages can be easily removed and submitted if required. The workbook includes the following:

CHAPTER EXERCISES

Chapters include a variety of exercises, such as short answer questions, which are taken from the chapter's learning outcomes; fill-in-the-blank and matching questions, which are taken from the key terms of the chapter; and multiple choice questions that reinforce the chapter content.

The chapter exercises are intended to help you study and better understand the information presented in the corresponding chapter of the textbook. Please take the time to work through them carefully. Answers to the workbook exercises are available through your instructor.

COMPETENCY SHEETS

A competency is the process that is used to evaluate the dental assistant's mastery of preclinical, clinical, administrative, and advanced skills. The competency sheets included within this workbook are designed to give you the opportunity to practice a skill until you have mastered it. There are spaces on the form that allow for at least three different evaluations: from yourself, from a peer, and from your instructor. The first time you perform a competency, you may wish to evaluate your own performance. The second time, you might ask a classmate to give you feedback. When you feel comfortable with that skill, the evaluator would be your instructor, clinic supervisor, or dentist.

FLASHCARDS

The flashcards in the back of this workbook are easily removed from the workbook to become a bonus study tool. Flashcards are made up of key information from the textbook about the sciences, medical emergencies, infection control, radiography, dental materials, instruments, and dental procedures to help you prepare for courses and for the certification exam.

We wish you success in your studies and in your chosen profession of dental assisting.

Debbie S. Robinson
Doni L. Bird

1 Introduction to Dental Assisting

TRUE/FALSE

_____ 1. Evidence of decay of human teeth has been found from the most ancient times.

_____ 2. The most important person in the dental practice is the patient.

_____ 3. The dental laboratory technician works only according to written prescription by the dental assistant.

_____ 4. The circulating dental assistant is used in four-handed dentistry.

_____ 5. A dental hygienist must pass both a written and a clinical examination to become licensed.

_____ 6. The clean area is where instruments are wrapped before sterilization.

_____ 7. The first dentist to use a dental assistant was Dr. C. Edmund Wells.

SHORT ANSWER

List the members of the dental health team.

8.

9.

10.

11.

12.

List the dental specialties.

13.

14.

15.

16.

17.

18.

19.

20.

21.

List and describe the different areas found in a dental office.

22.

23.

24.

25.

26.

27.

FILL IN THE BLANK

28. _____ is the specialty of diagnosis and surgical treatment of disorders, injuries, and defects of the oral and maxillofacial region.

29. _____ is the specialty of diagnosis and treatment of diseases of the supporting and surrounding tissues of the teeth.

30. _____ is the specialty of correction of all forms of malocclusion of the dentofacial structures.

31. _____ is the specialty of prevention and control of dental diseases and promotion of dental health through organized community efforts.

32. _____ is concerned with preventive and oral healthcare of children from birth through adolescence.

33. _____ is the specialty of diagnosis, prevention, and treatment of diseases and injuries of the pulp and associated tissues surrounding the root.

34. _____ is the specialty concerned with the nature of diseases affecting the oral structures and adjacent regions.

35. _____ is the specialty concerned with restoration and maintenance of oral functions by the restoration of natural teeth and/or replacement of missing teeth.

3

2 Professional and Legal Aspects of Dental Assisting

SHORT ANSWER

List three steps for good risk management.

1.

2.

3.

List three essential aspects of a professional appearance.

4.

5.

6.

List four personal qualities of a good dental assistant.

7.

8.

9.

10.

FILL IN THE BLANK

11. _____ is when the dentist is physically present in the office at the time the auxiliary performs certain functions.

12. _____ is codes of behavior, values, and morals.

13. _____ is the agency responsible for registration of disinfectants.

14. _____ is the organization that addresses issues of infection control.

15. The _____ issues clearances for all dental and medical devices.

16. _____ is when the dentist does not have to be physically present when the dental auxiliary performs certain functions.

17. _____ is the agency responsible for employee safety.

18. A statement made at the time of an alleged negligent act and that is admissible as evidence in a court of law is called _____.

MULTIPLE CHOICE QUESTIONS

19. Which of the following are correct regarding entries to the patient record?
    a. Write legibly in pencil.
    b. If there is an error, cover it with whiteout.
    c. Business and financial information must be included in the clinical record.
    d. None of the above

20. The patient's record should include notes about:
    a. treatment performed
    b. broken appointments
    c. last-minute cancellations
    d. all of the above

21. The dental assistant who performs "expanded functions" that are not allowed in his or her state is guilty of:
    a. the unlicensed practice of dentistry
    b. a breech of contract
    c. abandonment of the patient
    d. all of the above

22. Which of the following statements regarding ownership of dental records and radiographs are true?
    a. The dentist "owns" all patient records and radiographs.
    b. Patients have a right to review their records and radiographs.
    c. Original records and radiographs should never be allowed to leave the practice without the permission of the dentist.
    d. All of the above

Correcting a Chart Entry

Performance Objective

To correct an error on a patient's record.

Grading Criteria

3 Student meets most of the criteria without assistance.

2 Student requires assistance to meet the stated criteria.

1 Student did not prepare accordingly for the stated criteria.

0 Not applicable.

Criteria	Peer	Self	Instructor	Comment
1. Drew a single line through the previous entry.				
2. Initialed and dated the change.				
3. Wrote the correct entry on the next available line.				
4. Initialed and dated the new entry.				

Total amount of points earned _____

Grade _____ *Instructor's initials* _____

Chapter **2** **Professional and Legal Aspects of Dental Assisting**

3 Anatomy and Physiology

TRUE/FALSE

_____ 1. The midsagittal plane is the plane that divides the human body into equal left and right halves.

_____ 2. Cells are the smallest living unit of the body.

_____ 3. Tissues are groups of specialized cells that join together to perform a specific function.

_____ 4. A frenum is a narrow band of tissue that connects two bones.

_____ 5. The trigeminal nerve is the primary source of innervation for the oral cavity.

_____ 6. There are three types of muscle tissue.

_____ 7. The mandible forms the lower jaw and is the only movable bone of the skull.

_____ 8. The temporal process of the zygomatic bone forms the back of the skull.

_____ 9. The occipital bone forms the chin.

_____ 10. The frontal bone forms the forehead.

LABELING

11. Label the frontal view of the skull.

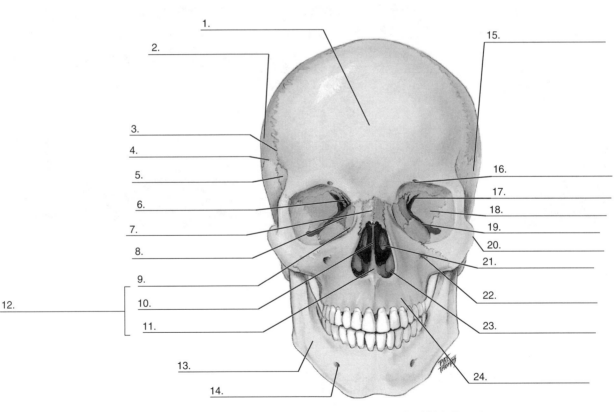

From Applegate E: The anatomy and physiology learning system, ed 3, St Louis, 2006, Saunders.

12. Label the bones and landmarks of the hard palate.

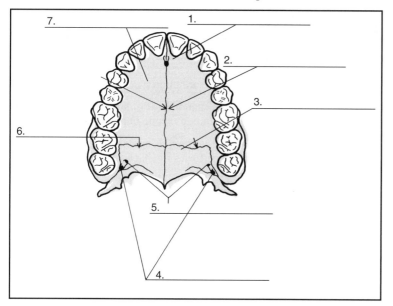

13. Identify each landmark by number.

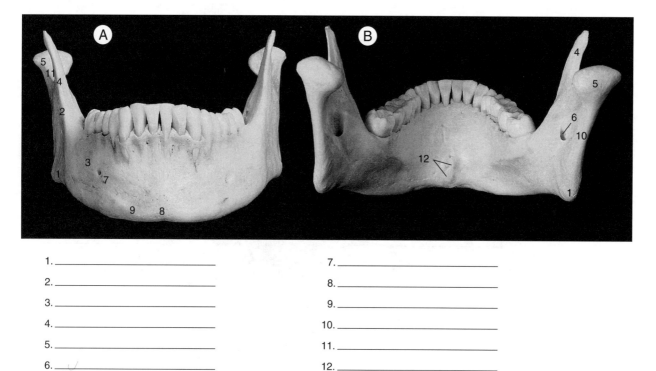

1. _____   7. _____

2. _____   8. _____

3. _____   9. _____

4. _____   10. _____

5. _____   11. _____

6. _____   12. _____

From Malamed S: Handbook of local anesthesia, ed 5, St Louis, 2004, Mosby.

14. Label the topical view of the mandible.

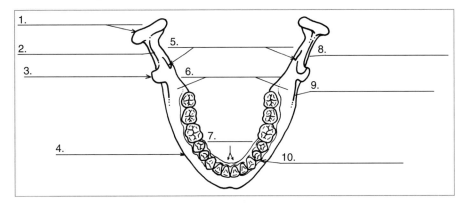

1. _____

2. _____

3. _____

5. _____

6. _____

7. _____

4. _____

8. _____

9. _____

10. _____

Identifying the Major Landmarks and Structures of the Face

Performance Objective

The student will be able to identify the major landmarks and structures of the face.

Grading Criteria

3 Student meets most of the criteria without assistance.

2 Student requires assistance to meet the stated criteria.

1 Student did not prepare accordingly for the stated criteria.

0 Not applicable.

Criteria	Peer	Self	Instructor	Comment
1. Identified the ala of the nose.				
2. Identified the inner canthus and outer canthus of the eye.				
3. Identified the commissure of the lips.				
4. Identified the location of the frontal sinuses.				
5. Identified the location of the maxillary sinuses.				
6. Identified the location of the parotid glands.				
7. Identified the philtrum.				
8. Identified the tragus of the ear.				
9. Identified the vermilion border.				
10. Identified the zygomatic arch.				

Total amount of points earned _____

Grade _____ *Instructor's initials* _____

Identifying the Major Landmarks, Structures, and Normal Tissues of the Mouth

Performance Objective

The student will be able to correctly identify the major landmarks, structures, and normal tissues of the mouth.

Grading Criteria

3 Student meets most of the criteria without assistance.

2 Student requires assistance to meet the stated criteria.

1 Student did not prepare accordingly for the stated criteria.

0 Not applicable.

Criteria	Peer	Self	Instructor	Comment
1. Identified the dorsum of the tongue.				
2. Identified the area of the gag reflex.				
3. Identified the hard and soft palates.				
4. Identified the gingival margin.				
5. Identified the incisive papilla.				
6. Identified the mandibular labial frenum.				
7. Identified the maxillary labial frenum.				
8. Identified the sublingual frenum.				
9. Identified the vestibule of the mouth.				
10. Identified Wharton's duct.				

Total amount of points earned _____

Grade _____ *Instructor's initials* _____

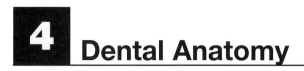

Dental Anatomy

TRUE/FALSE

_____ 1. The clinical crown is that portion of the tooth that is visible in the mouth.

_____ 2. In the permanent dentition, there are 12 molar teeth.

_____ 3. An embrasure is the space between the roots of a molar.

_____ 4. Primary teeth are also known as deciduous teeth.

_____ 5. The anatomic crown is that portion of the tooth that is covered with enamel.

_____ 6. Bifurcation means division into three roots.

_____ 7. Molars and premolars have incisal surfaces.

_____ 8. Dentin makes up the main portion of the tooth structure.

_____ 9. Cementum is harder than enamel or dentin.

_____ 10. Only posterior teeth have periodontal ligaments.

LABELING

11. Label the tissues of the tooth and surrounding structures.

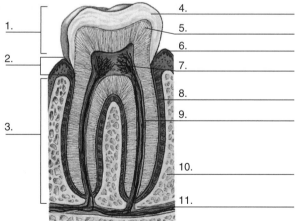

12. Identify the types of tooth contour.

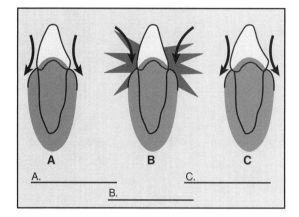

A. _____   C. _____

B. _____

13. Label the portions of the dental pulp.

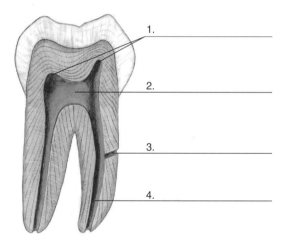

Identifying the Teeth and Naming the Tooth Surfaces

Performance Objective

The student will be able to correctly identify the teeth and name the tooth surfaces.

Grading Criteria

3 Student meets most of the criteria without assistance.

2 Student requires assistance to meet the stated criteria.

1 Student did not prepare accordingly for the stated criteria.

0 Not applicable.

Criteria	Peer	Self	Instructor	Comment
1. Identified the surfaces of the maxillary central incisors.				
2. Identified the surfaces of the mandibular central incisors.				
3. Identified the surfaces of the maxillary lateral incisors.				
4. Identified the surfaces of the mandibular lateral incisors.				
5. Identified the surfaces of the maxillary canines.				
6. Identified the surfaces of the mandibular canines.				
7. Identified the surfaces of the maxillary premolars.				
8. Identified the surfaces of the mandibular premolars.				
9. Identified the surfaces of the maxillary molars.				
10. Identified the surfaces of the mandibular molars.				
11. Identified the occlusal surfaces.				
12. Identified the incisal surfaces.				
13. Identified the lingual surfaces.				
14. Identified the facial surfaces.				
15. Identified the mesial surface of the maxillary central incisors.				
16. Identified the distal surface of the mandibular central incisors.				

Total amount of points earned _____

Grade _____ *Instructor's initials* _____

Identifying the Primary and Permanent Dentition Using the Universal, Federation Dentaire Internationale, and Palmer Notation Numbering Systems

Performance Objective

The student will be able to correctly identify the primary and permanent dentition using the Universal, Federation Dentaire Internationale, and Palmer Notation Numbering Systems.

Grading Criteria

3 Student meets most of the criteria without assistance.

2 Student requires assistance to meet the stated criteria.

1 Student did not prepare accordingly for the stated criteria.

0 Not applicable.

Criteria	Peer	Self	Instructor	Comment
1. Identified the primary teeth in each arch using the Universal Numbering System.				
2. Identified the primary teeth in each arch using the Federation Dentaire Internationale Numbering System.				
3. Identified the primary teeth in each arch using the Palmer Notation Numbering System.				
4. Identified the permanent teeth in each arch using the Universal Numbering System.				
5. Identified the permanent teeth in each arch using the Federation Dentaire Internationale Numbering System.				
6. Identified the permanent teeth in each arch using the Palmer Notation Numbering System.				

Total amount of points earned _____

Grade _____ *Instructor's initials* _____

5 | Disease Transmission

TRUE/FALSE

_____ 1. A pathogen is a microorganism that is not capable of causing disease.

_____ 2. Many types of bacteria are actually beneficial to humans.

_____ 3. When bacteria are in the spore state, they cannot cause disease.

_____ 4. Viruses are much larger in size than bacteria.

_____ 5. Virulence describes the ability of a pathogen to cause disease.

_____ 6. An acute infection is of short duration.

_____ 7. Indirect transmission of disease is also known as cross contamination.

_____ 8. Diseases cannot be transmitted during a dental procedure through aerosol or spray.

_____ 9. Airborne disease transmission is also known as droplet infection.

_____ 10. The term parenteral transmission refers to disease spread from parent to child.

FILL IN THE BLANK

11. The number of pathogens present is called the _____.

12. _____ is a disease caused by a spore-forming bacillus.

13. The ability of the human body to resist disease is called _____.

14. The method by which the pathogen enters the body is called the _____.

15. Plants such as mushroom, yeasts, and molds are examples of _____.

16. _____ is a disease of the liver with a latency of up to 15 to 25 years.

17. _____ is a disease of the liver caused by fecal-oral transmission.

18. _____ is a type of disease caused by normally nonpathogenic organisms.

19. _____ is a disease caused by the yeast *Candida albicans*.

20. _____ transmission occurs through a break in the skin.

MULTIPLE CHOICE

21. Which of the following organisms live and multiply only inside a host cell?
    a. bacteria
    b. virus
    c. spore
    d. all of the above

22. The ability of the human body to resist a pathogen is called _____.
    a. latency
    b. host resistance
    c. link of transmission
    d. portal of entry

23. Which of the following surfaces could be a potential source of disease transmission in a dental office?
    a. faucets
    b. instrument drawer handles
    c. dental materials
    d. the patient's chart
    e. all of the above

24. Dental aerosols can contain _____.
    a. saliva
    b. blood
    c. microorganisms
    d. all of the above

25. Which of the following are considered types of parenteral disease transmission?
    a. needlesticks
    b. human bites
    c. cuts
    d. all of the above

6 Infection Control and Management of Hazardous Materials

TRUE/FALSE

_____ 1. The Centers for Disease Control and Prevention (CDC) is not a regulatory agency.

_____ 2. OSHA's Bloodborne Pathogen Standard (BBP) is the most important infection-control law in dentistry.

_____ 3. The concept of "universal precautions" has been expanded, and the term for the new concept is "standard precautions."

_____ 4. A category III employee is routinely exposed to blood, saliva, or both.

_____ 5. The employer is not required to offer the hepatitis B vaccine to category III employees.

_____ 6. You should always bend or break needles before disposal.

_____ 7. The sharps container must be labeled with the biohazard symbol.

_____ 8. Alcohol-based hand rubs are not to be used if your hands are visibly soiled.

_____ 9. Artificial nails should not be worn by dental assistants.

_____ 10. Short sleeve scrub tops are adequate protection when assisting with procedures.

FILL IN THE BLANK

11. A category _____ employee is one who is routinely exposed to blood and/or saliva.

12. Employers are required by the _____ _____ Standard to provide employees with personal protective equipment.

13. A _____ is an acceptable alternative to eyewear.

14. _____ gloves are required for surgical procedures.

15. _____ gloves should be worn when disinfecting surfaces in the treatment room.

MULTIPLE CHOICE

16. The term "medical waste" refers to:
    a. contaminated waste
    b. infectious waste
    c. regulated waste
    d. all of the above

17. Which of the following must be included in a hazard communication program?
    a. written program
    b. inventory of hazardous chemicals
    c. MSDS for every chemical
    d. employee training
    e. all of the above

18. When using the National Fire Protection Association Labels, the blue diamond refers to what type of hazard?
    a. fire
    b. health
    c. reactivity
    d. all of the above

19. How long must employee training records in Hazard Communication be kept?
    a. 1 year
    b. 3 years
    c. 5 years
    d. indefinitely

20. Which of the following are bloodborne pathogens?
    a. hepatitis B
    b. hepatitis C
    c. HIV
    d. all of the above

Applying First Aid After an Exposure Incident

Performance Objective

The student will role-play the proper technique for first aid following an exposure incident.

Grading Criteria

3 Student meets most of the criteria without assistance.

2 Student requires assistance to meet the stated criteria.

1 Student did not prepare accordingly for the stated criteria.

0 Not applicable.

Criteria	Peer	Self	Instructor	Comment
1. Stopped operations immediately.				
2. Removed gloves.				
3. If the area of broken skin was bleeding, gently squeezed the site to express a small amount of visible blood.				
4. Washed hands thoroughly, using antimicrobial soap and warm water.				
5. Dried hands.				
6. Applied a small amount of antiseptic to the affected area.				
7. Applied an adhesive bandage to the area.				
8. Completed applicable postexposure follow-up steps.				
9. Notified the employer of the injury immediately after first aid was provided.				

Total amount of points earned _____

Grade _____ *Instructor's initials* _____

Performance Objective

The student will demonstrate the proper technique for handwashing before gloving.

Grading Criteria

3 Student meets most of the criteria without assistance.

2 Student requires assistance to meet the stated criteria.

1 Student did not prepare accordingly for the stated criteria.

0 Not applicable.

Criteria	Peer	Self	Instructor	Comment
1. Removed all jewelry, including watch and rings.				
2. Used the foot or electronic control to regulate the flow of water. (If this was not available, used a paper towel to grasp the faucets to turn them on and off. Discarded the towel after use.)				
3. Used liquid soap, dispensed with a foot-activated or electronic device.				
4. Vigorously rubbed lathered hands together under a stream of water to remove surface debris.				
5. Dispensed additional soap and vigorously rubbed lathered hands together for a minimum of 10 seconds under a stream of water.				
6. Rinsed the hands with cool water.				
7. Used a paper towel to thoroughly dry the hands and then the forearms.				

Total amount of points earned _____

Grade _____ *Instructor's initials* _____

Chapter **6** **Infection Control and Management of Hazardous Materials**

Applying an Alcohol-Based Hand Rub

Performance Objective

The student will demonstrate the proper technique for applying an alcohol-based hand rub.

Grading Criteria

3 Student meets most of the criteria without assistance.

2 Student requires assistance to meet the stated criteria.

1 Student did not prepare accordingly for the stated criteria.

0 Not applicable.

Criteria	Peer	Self	Instructor	Comment
1. Washed and dried hands thoroughly with soap and water if they were visibly soiled or contaminated with organic matter.				
2. Read the directions carefully to determine the proper amount of product to dispense.				
3. Dispensed the proper amount of the product into the palm of one hand.				
4. Rubbed the palms of the hands together.				
5. Rubbed the product in between the fingers.				
6. Rubbed the product over the back of the hands.				

Total amount of points earned _____

Grade _____ *Instructor's initials* _____

Putting on Personal Protective Equipment

Performance Objective

The student will demonstrate the proper technique for putting on personal protective equipment before patient care.

Grading Criteria

3 Student meets most of the criteria without assistance.

2 Student requires assistance to meet the stated criteria.

1 Student did not prepare accordingly for the stated criteria.

0 Not applicable.

Criteria	Peer	Self	Instructor	Comment
1. Put on protective clothing over the uniform, street clothes, or scrubs.				
2. Put on a surgical mask and adjusted the fit.				
3. Put on protective eyewear.				
4. Thoroughly washed and dried the hands. (If hands were not visibly soiled, used an alcohol-based hand rub.)				
5. Held one glove at the cuff, placed the opposite hand inside the glove, and pulled it onto the hand. Repeated the procedure with a new glove for the other hand.				

Note: The sequence of Nos. 2 and 3 may be interchangeable. Most important is that the gloves are put on last to prevent contaminating them before they are placed in the patient's mouth.

Total amount of points earned _____

Grade _____ *Instructor's initials* _____

Removing Personal Protective Equipment

Performance Objective

The student will demonstrate the proper technique for removing personal protective equipment.

Grading Criteria

3 Student meets most of the criteria without assistance.

2 Student requires assistance to meet the stated criteria.

1 Student did not prepare accordingly for the stated criteria.

0 Not applicable.

Criteria	Peer	Self	Instructor	Comment
Protective Clothing				
1. Pulled the gown off, turning it inside out during removal.				
2. Ensured that the contaminated outside surface of the gown did not touch underlying clothes or skin during removal.				
Gloves				
1. Used a gloved hand to grasp the opposite glove at the outside cuff. Pulled downward, turning the glove inside out while pulling it away from the hand.				
2. For the other hand, used ungloved fingers to grasp the inside (uncontaminated area) of the cuff of the remaining glove. Pulled downward to remove the glove, turning it inside out.				
3. Discarded the gloves into the waste receptacle.				
4. Washed and thoroughly dried hands. *Note: If no visible contamination exists and if gloves have not been torn or punctured during the procedure, an alcohol-based hand rub may be used in place of handwashing.*				
Eyewear				
1. Removed the eyewear by touching it only on the ear rests.				
2. Placed the eyewear on a disposable towel for proper cleaning and disinfecting.				
Masks				
1. Slid fingers on each hand under the elastic strap in front of ears and removed the mask, ensuring that fingers contacted only the mask's ties or elastic strap.				
2. Discarded the mask into the waste receptacle.				

Total amount of points earned _____

Grade _____ *Instructor's initials* _____

Creating an Appropriate Label for a Secondary Container

Performance Objective

The student will demonstrate the proper technique for using information from a Material Safety Data Sheet (MSDS) to complete a chemical label for a secondary container.

Grading Criteria

3 Student meets most of the criteria without assistance.

2 Student requires assistance to meet the stated criteria.

1 Student did not prepare accordingly for the stated criteria.

0 Not applicable.

Criteria	Peer	Self	Instructor	Comment
1. Wrote the manufacturer's name and address on the label.				
2. Wrote the name of the chemical(s) on the label.				
3. Wrote the appropriate health hazard code in the blue triangle.				
4. Wrote the appropriate flammability and explosion hazard code in the red triangle.				
5. Wrote the appropriate reactivity code in the yellow triangle.				
6. Wrote the appropriate specific hazard warning in the white triangle.				

Total amount of points earned _____

Grade _____ *Instructor's initials* _____

7 Surface Disinfection and Treatment Room Preparation

TRUE/FALSE

_____ 1. The purpose of surface barriers is to prevent contamination.

_____ 2. Treatment surfaces can be disinfected without precleaning if there is no visible blood.

_____ 3. Utility gloves should be worn when precleaning surfaces.

_____ 4. Surfaces that are smooth and easily accessible are the easiest to clean and disinfect.

_____ 5. Precleaning is done after the disinfection process.

_____ 6. Blood and saliva are also known as bioburden.

_____ 7. If a surface is not clean, it can be easily disinfected.

_____ 8. Surface barriers should be resistant to fluids.

_____ 9. There is a wide variety of types of barriers.

_____ 10. Not all types of disinfectants contain a precleaning agent.

FILL IN THE BLANK

11. A forceps is classified as a _____ type of instrument.

12. An x-ray PID is classified as a _____ type of instrument.

13. A _____ is a chemical that is used on skin.

14. An amalgam carrier is classified as a _____ type of instrument.

15. A chemical that is used on hard surfaces or instruments is a _____.

MULTIPLE CHOICE

16. Which of the following can be used as surface barriers?
    a. plastic bags
    b. aluminum foil
    c. plastic sticky tape
    d. all of the above

17. Which agency registers surface disinfectants?
    a. Environmental Protection Agency (EPA)
    b. Occupational Safety and Health Administration (OSHA)
    c. Food and Drug Administration (FDA)
    d. all of the above

18. Which of the following disinfectants can cause red or yellow stains?
    a. synthetic phenols
    b. iodophors
    c. sodium hypochlorite
    d. none of the above

19. Which of the following are disadvantages of alcohol as a disinfectant?
    a. rapid evaporation
    b. not effective in the presence of bioburden
    c. damaging to plastics and vinyls
    d. all of the above

20. Which of the following can be used as a high-level disinfectant or a sterilant?
    a. alcohol
    b. synthetic phenol
    c. glutaraldehyde
    d. all of the above

Placing and Removing Surface Barriers

Performance Objective

The student will demonstrate the proper technique for placing and removing surface barriers.

Grading Criteria

3 Student meets most of the criteria without assistance.

2 Student requires assistance to meet the stated criteria.

1 Student did not prepare accordingly for the stated criteria.

0 Not applicable.

Criteria	Peer	Self	Instructor	Comment
Placement of Surface Barriers				
1. Washed and dried hands.				
2. Assembled the appropriate setup.				
3. Selected the appropriate surface barriers.				
4. Placed each barrier over the entire surface to be protected.				
Removal of Surface Barriers				
1. Wore utility gloves to remove contaminated surface barriers.				
2. Very carefully removed each cover.				
3. Discarded the used covers into the regular waste receptacle.				
4. Washed, disinfected, and removed utility gloves.				
5. Washed and dried hands.				

Total amount of points earned _____

Grade _____ *Instructor's initials* _____

Performing Treatment Room Cleaning and Disinfection

Performance Objective

The student will demonstrate the proper technique for precleaning and disinfecting a dental treatment room and equipment surfaces.

Grading Criteria

3 Student meets most of the criteria without assistance.

2 Student requires assistance to meet the stated criteria.

1 Student did not prepare accordingly for the stated criteria.

0 Not applicable.

Criteria	Peer	Self	Instructor	Comment
1. Assembled the appropriate setup.				
2. Wore the appropriate personal protective eyewear.				
3. Checked to see that the precleaning-disinfecting product had been prepared correctly and was fresh. Read and followed the manufacturer's instructions.				
4. Sprayed the paper towel or gauze pad with the product and vigorously wiped the surface.				
5. Sprayed a fresh paper towel or gauze pad with the product.				
6. Allowed the surface to remain moist for the manufacturer's recommended time.				

Total amount of points earned _____

Grade _____ *Instructor's initials* _____

Disinfecting an Alginate Impression

Performance Objective

The student will demonstrate the proper technique for disinfecting an alginate impression.

Grading Criteria

3 Student meets most of the criteria without assistance.

2 Student requires assistance to meet the stated criteria.

1 Student did not prepare accordingly for the stated criteria.

0 Not applicable.

Criteria	Peer	Self	Instructor	Comment
1. Assembled the appropriate setup.				
2. Wore the appropriate personal protective eyewear.				
3. Gently cleaned the impression.				
4. Rinsed the impression and removed excess water.				
5. Sprayed the impression thoroughly with disinfectant.				
6. Wrapped the impression loosely in a plastic bag for the recommended contact time.				
7. After the sufficient contact time, rinsed the impression.				

Total amount of points earned _____

Grade _____ Instructor's initials _____

Instrument Processing

TRUE/FALSE

_____ 1. The ideal instrument processing area should be dedicated only to instrument processing.

_____ 2. An advantage of dry heat sterilization is that there is no corrosion on the instruments.

_____ 3. The size and shape of instrument processing areas are the same in all dental offices.

_____ 4. The container of the holding solution should be labeled with a biohazard label and a chemical label.

_____ 5. Soiled and clean instruments may be stored in the same cabinet.

SHORT ANSWER

List the seven steps in instrument processing.

6.

7.

8.

9.

10.

11.

12.

List three advantages of steam autoclave.

13.

14.

15.

FILL IN THE BLANK

16. _____ is the least desirable method of cleaning instruments.

17. A _____ prevents blood and debris from drying on the instrument.

18. A _____ loosens and removes debris from instruments.

19. A _____ sterilizes by super heated steam under pressure.

20. An automated washing and disinfecting machine is called a _____.

Operating the Ultrasonic Cleaner

Performance Objective

When provided with the appropriate materials, the student will demonstrate the proper technique for precleaning instruments before sterilization using the ultrasonic cleaner.

Grading Criteria

3 Student meets most of the criteria without assistance.

2 Student requires assistance to meet the stated criteria.

1 Student did not prepare accordingly for the stated criteria.

0 Not applicable.

Criteria	Peer	Self	Instructor	Comment
1. Wore appropriate personal protective eyewear.				
2. Removed the lid from the container and checked the level of solution.				
3. Placed instruments or cassette into the basket.				
4. Replaced the lid and turned the cycle to ON.				
5. After the cleaning cycle, removed the basket and rinsed the instruments.				
6. Emptied the basket onto the towel.				
7. Replaced the lid on the ultrasonic cleaner.				

Total amount of points earned _____

Grade _____ *Instructor's initials* _____

Autoclaving Instruments

Performance Objective

When provided with the appropriate materials, the student will demonstrate the proper technique for preparing and autoclaving instruments.

Grading Criteria

3 Student meets most of the criteria without assistance.

2 Student requires assistance to meet the stated criteria.

1 Student did not prepare accordingly for the stated criteria.

0 Not applicable.

Criteria	Peer	Self	Instructor	Comment
1. Wore appropriate personal protective eyewear.				
2. Dried the instruments.				
3. Dipped nonstainless instruments and burs in a corrosion inhibitor.				
4. Placed the process indicator into the package.				
5. Packaged, sealed, and labeled the instruments.				
6. Placed, bagged, and sealed items in the autoclave.				
7. Tilted glass or metal canisters at an angle.				
8. Placed larger packs at the bottom of the chamber.				
9. Did not overload the autoclave.				
10. Followed the manufacturer's instructions.				
11. Checked the level of water. (If necessary, added additional distilled water.)				
12. Set the autoclave controls for the appropriate time, temperature, and pressure.				
13. At the end of the sterilization cycle, vented the steam into the room, and allowed the contents of the autoclave to dry and cool.				
14. Checked the external process indicator for color change.				
15. Removed the instruments when they were cool and dry.				

Total amount of points earned _____

Grade _____ *Instructor's initials* _____

Sterilizing Instruments With Chemical Vapor

Performance Objective

When provided with the appropriate materials, the student will demonstrate the proper technique for preparing and sterilizing instruments with chemical vapor.

Grading Criteria

3 Student meets most of the criteria without assistance.

2 Student requires assistance to meet the stated criteria.

1 Student did not prepare accordingly for the stated criteria.

0 Not applicable.

Criteria	Peer	Self	Instructor	Comment
1. Wore appropriate personal protective eyewear.				
2. Dried the instruments.				
3. Wrapped the instruments.				
4. Ensured that packages were not too large.				
5. Read and followed the manufacturer's instructions.				
6. Read the information on the MSDS for the chemical liquid.				
7. Loaded the sterilizer.				
8. Set the controls for the proper time and temperature.				
9. Followed the manufacturer's instructions for venting and cooling.				
10. Checked the external process indicator for color change.				
11. Removed the instruments when they were cool and dry.				

Total amount of points earned _____

Grade _____ *Instructor's initials* _____

Sterilizing Instruments With Dry Heat

Performance Objective

When provided with the appropriate materials, the student will demonstrate the proper technique for preparing and sterilizing instruments with dry heat.

Grading Criteria

3 Student meets most of the criteria without assistance.

2 Student requires assistance to meet the stated criteria.

1 Student did not prepare accordingly for the stated criteria.

0 Not applicable.

Criteria	Peer	Self	Instructor	Comment
1. Wore appropriate personal protective eyewear.				
2. Dried the instruments before wrapping.				
3. Opened hinged instruments.				
4. Wrapped instruments.				
5. Read and followed the manufacturer's instructions.				
6. Loaded the instruments into the dry heat chamber.				
7. Set the time and temperature.				
8. Did not place additional instruments in the load once the sterilization cycle had begun.				
9. Allowed the packs to cool before handling.				
10. Checked the indicators for color change.				

Total amount of points earned _____

Grade _____ *Instructor's initials* _____

Performance Objective

When provided with the appropriate materials, the student will demonstrate the proper technique for preparing and sterilizing instruments with a chemical sterilant.

Grading Criteria

3 Student meets most of the criteria without assistance.

2 Student requires assistance to meet the stated criteria.

1 Student did not prepare accordingly for the stated criteria.

0 Not applicable.

Criteria	Peer	Self	Instructor	Comment
Preparing the Solution				
1. Wore utility gloves, a mask, eyewear, and protective clothing when preparing, using, and discarding the solution.				
2. Followed the manufacturer's instructions for preparing and/or activating, using, and disposing of the solution.				
3. Prepared the solution for use as a sterilant. Labeled the containers with the name of the chemical, date of preparation, and any other information relating to the hazards of the product.				
4. Covered the container and kept it closed unless putting instruments in or taking them out.				
Using the Solution				
1. Precleaned, rinsed, and dried items to be processed.				
2. Placed the items in a perforated tray or pan. Placed the pan in the solution and covered the container. Or as an alternative, used tongs.				
3. Ensured that all items were fully submerged in the solution for the entire contact time.				
4. Rinsed processed items thoroughly with water and dried. Placed items in a clean package.				
Maintaining the Solution				
1. Tested the glutaraldehyde concentration of the solution with a chemical test kit (available from the manufacturer).				
2. Replaced the solution as indicated on the instructions or when the level of the solution became low or visibly dirty.				
3. When replacing the used solution, discarded all of the used solution, cleaned the container with a detergent, rinsed with water, dried, and filled the container with fresh solution.				

Total amount of points earned _____

Grade _____ *Instructor's initials* _____

Performance Objective

The student will demonstrate the proper technique for performing biologic monitoring.

Grading Criteria

3 Student meets most of the criteria without assistance.

2 Student requires assistance to meet the stated criteria.

1 Student did not prepare accordingly for the stated criteria.

0 Not applicable.

Criteria	Peer	Self	Instructor	Comment
1. While wearing all PPE, placed the BI strip in the bundle of instruments and sealed the package.				
2. Placed the pack with the BI strip in the center of the sterilizer load.				
3. Placed the remainder of the packaged instruments into the sterilizer and processed the load through a normal sterilization cycle.				
4. Removed utility gloves, mask, and eyewear. Washed and dried hands.				
5. Recorded the date of the test, the type of sterilizer, the cycle, temperature, time, and the name of the person operating the sterilizer.				
6. Removed and processed BI strip after the load was sterilized.				
7. Mailed the processed spore test strips and the control BI strip to the monitoring service.				

Total amount of points earned _____

Grade _____ *Instructor's initials* _____

9 Clinical Dentistry

TRUE/FALSE

_____ 1. The dental treatment area can also be referred to as the dental ambulatory center.

_____ 2. A standard routine procedure must be followed when admitting and positioning the patient and dental team.

_____ 3. The patient's personal items should be handed to the front desk staff for safekeeping during a procedure.

_____ 4. In a subsupine position, the patient's head is actually lower than their feet.

_____ 5. The science that seeks to adapt working conditions to suit workers is ergonomics.

_____ 6. For correct operator positioning, the operator should be positioned approximately 4 to 5 inches higher than the assistant.

_____ 7. Problems associated with continued flexion and extension of the wrist is carpal tunnel syndrome.

_____ 8. An instrument is exchanged from the assistant to the dentist in the transfer zone.

_____ 9. At the beginning of a procedure, the operator will use the mouth mirror and air-water syringe to inspect the area to be treated.

_____ 10. The dental assistant uses their left hand to transfer instruments while holding the oral evacuation system in their right hand.

MATCHING

Match the following dental treatment equipment to its description.

_____ 11. Dental chair

_____ 12. Curing light

_____ 13. Dental unit

_____ 14. Operator's stool

_____ 15. Oral evacuation

_____ 16. Operating light

_____ 17. Assistant's stool

_____ 18. Air-water syringe

_____ 19. Amalgamator

A. Illuminates the oral cavity

B. Designed to support the patient comfortably

C. Provides stability, mobility, and comfort for the assistant

D. Provides the electricity and air to equipment

E. Used to rinse or dry areas of the mouth

F. To support the operator for long periods of time

G. Triturates encapsulated dental materials

H. Removes fluids and debris from the mouth

I. Activates the polymerization of resins and composites

SHORT ANSWER

20. Describe the four goals the dental assistant and dentist should work closely together to accomplish.

21. List the specific criteria for proper positioning of the seated operator.

22. List the specific criteria for proper positioning of the seated dental assistant.

23. Name the three types of operator grasps commonly used when receiving an instrument.

LABELING

24. Using the diagram below, label each zone, and describe what should be in each of those areas.

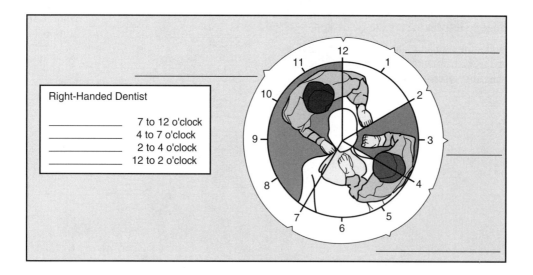

Right-Handed Dentist

_____ 7 to 12 o'clock
_____ 4 to 7 o'clock
_____ 2 to 4 o'clock
_____ 12 to 2 o'clock

Admitting and Seating the Patient

Performance Objective

The student will admit, seat, and prepare the patient for treatment.

Grading Criteria

3 Student meets most of the criteria without assistance.

2 Student requires assistance to meet the stated criteria.

1 Student did not prepare accordingly for the stated criteria.

0 Not applicable.

Criteria	Peer	Self	Instructor	Comment
1. Ensured that the treatment room was properly cleaned and prepared, with the chair properly positioned and the patient's path clear.				
2. Placed instrument setup and materials out.				
3. Identified and greeted the patient accordingly.				
4. Escorted the patient to the treatment area.				
5. Placed the patient's personal items in a safe place in the treatment room.				
6. Properly seated the patient.				
7. Placed the patient's napkin around the neck.				
8. Properly positioned the dental chair for the procedure.				
9. Adjusted the operating light and then turned it on.				
10. Maintained patient comfort throughout these preparations.				

Total amount of points earned _____

Grade _____ *Instructor's initials* _____

Transferring Instruments Using the Single-Handed and Two-Handed Techniques

Performance Objective

The student will perform single-handed and specialized instrument transfer in a safe and efficient manner.

Grading Criteria

3 Student meets most of the criteria without assistance.

2 Student requires assistance to meet the stated criteria.

1 Student did not prepare accordingly for the stated criteria.

0 Not applicable.

Criteria	Peer	Self	Instructor	Comment
Single-Handed Transfer and Exchange				
1. Retrieved the instrument from the instrument tray opposite the working end.				
2. Held the instrument in the transfer zone, 8 to 10 inches away from the dentist.				
3. Anticipated the dentist's transfer signal and positioned the new instrument parallel to the instrument in the dentist's hand.				
4. Retrieved the used instrument using the last two fingers.				
5. Delivered the new instrument to the dentist.				
6. Maintained safety throughout the transfer.				
Nonlocking Cotton Pliers Transfer				
1. Held the contents (cotton pellet) securely by pinching the beaks together.				
2. Delivered the pliers so the dentist could hold the beaks together.				
3. Retrieved the pliers without dropping the cotton pellet.				
Forceps Transfer				
1. Used the right hand to pick up the forceps and hold it for delivery in the position of use.				
2. Used the left hand to retrieve the used instrument from the dentist.				
3. Delivered the new instrument to the dentist in the appropriate position.				
4. Returned the used instrument to its proper position on the tray.				

Criteria	Peer	Self	Instructor	Comment
Handpiece Exchange				
1. Used the left hand to pick up the handpiece and hold it for delivery in the position of use.				
2. Used the right hand to take the used instrument from the dentist.				
3. Delivered the handpiece to the dentist in the appropriate position.				
4. When exchanging two handpieces, did not tangle the cords.				
Air-Water Syringe Transfer				
1. Held the nozzle of the air-water syringe in the delivery fingers.				
2. Retrieved the instrument the dentist was using, then delivered the syringe.				
Scissors Transfer				
1. Picked up the scissors and held them near the working end with the beaks slightly open.				
2. Positioned the handle of the scissors over the dentist's fingers.				
3. Retrieved the used instrument with the right hand.				

Total amount of points earned _____

Grade _____ *Instructor's initials* _____

10 Moisture Control

TRUE/FALSE

_____ 1. A dry-angle is a triangle-shaped absorbent pad to help isolate anterior areas of the mouth.

_____ 2. The anchor tooth is the tooth that holds the dental dam clamp.

_____ 3. When working on the posterior area of the maxillary arch, a cotton roll is placed on the cheek side.

_____ 4. A limited-area rinse should only be performed at the completion of the dental procedure.

_____ 5. The oral evacuator may be held in either the thumb to nose grasp or the palm grasp.

_____ 6. HVE is the abbreviation for high-volume evacuator.

_____ 7. The isolation technique that can ensure dry conditions is the dental dam.

_____ 8. HVE tips should be disinfected after use.

_____ 9. A system used to remove small amounts of saliva or water from a patient's mouth is the saliva ejector.

_____ 10. The dental dam is applied before the local anesthetic is administered.

MATCHING

_____ 11. Dental dam punch

_____ 12. Dental dam stamp

_____ 13. Dental dam

_____ 14. Dental dam forceps

_____ 15. Dental dam frame

_____ 16. Dental dam clamps

_____ 17. Dental dam napkin

_____ 18. Lubricant

A. U-shaped piece of equipment to stretch the dam away from the face

B. Used to place and remove the dental dam clamp

C. Device used to create holes in the dam

D. Disposable absorbent placed between the face and dam

E. Device used to mark teeth on the dam

F. Material used to isolate teeth

G. Water-soluble substance placed on the underside of the dam

H. Piece of metal that anchors the dental dam material on the tooth

SHORT ANSWER

19. List the three uses of the high-volume evacuator.

20. Describe the advantages and disadvantages of cotton rolls.

21. Below are locations of handpiece placement during a procedure for a right-handed operator. Fill in the surface of each tooth on which you would position the HVE tip.

If handpiece placement is on:	The HVE should be positioned on:
a. Facial surface of #9	_____
b. Occlusal surface of #4	_____
c. Lingual surface of #18	_____
d. Occlusal surface of #13	_____
e. Lingual surface of #24	_____
f. Buccal surface of #30	_____

22. List the indications for using the dental dam.

Performance Objective

The student will perform a limited-area rinse and a complete mouth rinse using the high-volume oral evacuator (HVE) and air-water syringe.

Grading Criteria

3 Student meets most of the criteria without assistance.

2 Student requires assistance to meet the stated criteria.

1 Student did not prepare accordingly for the stated criteria.

0 Not applicable.

Criteria	Peer	Self	Instructor	Comment
Limited-Area Rinse				
1. Held the air-water syringe in the left hand.				
2. Held the HVE in the right hand using a proper grasp.				
3. Positioned the HVE in the operative site then rinsed and suctioned the area.				
4. Maintained patient comfort and followed appropriate infection-control measures throughout the procedure.				
Complete Mouth Rinse				
1. Held the air-water syringe in the left hand.				
2. Held the HVE in the right hand using a proper grasp.				
3. Positioned the HVE in the vestibule of the mouth and, starting at one area, rinsed the mouth thoroughly, suctioning the accumulated water and debris.				
4. Maintained patient comfort and followed appropriate infection-control measures throughout the procedure.				

Total amount of points earned _____

Grade _____ *Instructor's initials* _____

Performance Objective

The student will maintain moisture control, access, and visibility during patient care by appropriately positioning the high-volume oral evacuator (HVE).

Grading Criteria

3 Student meets most of the criteria without assistance.

2 Student requires assistance to meet the stated criteria.

1 Student did not prepare accordingly for the stated criteria.

0 Not applicable.

Criteria	Peer	Self	Instructor	Comment
1. Assumed the correct seated position to accommodate a left-handed or right-handed dentist.				
2. Used the proper grasp when holding the HVE.				
3. Grasped the air-water syringe in the left hand during HVE placement.				
4. Positioned the HVE correctly for the maxillary left posterior treatment.				
5. Positioned the HVE correctly for the maxillary right posterior treatment.				
6. Positioned the HVE correctly for the mandibular left posterior treatment.				
7. Positioned the HVE correctly for the mandibular right posterior treatment.				
8. Positioned the HVE correctly for the anterior treatment with lingual access.				
9. Positioned the HVE correctly for the anterior treatment with facial access.				
10. Maintained patient comfort and followed appropriate infection-control measures throughout the procedure.				

Total amount of points earned _____

Grade _____ *Instructor's initials* _____

Placing and Removing Cotton Rolls

Performance Objective

The student will place and properly remove cotton roll isolation for each area of the mouth.

Grading Criteria

3 Student meets most of the criteria without assistance.

2 Student requires assistance to meet the stated criteria.

1 Student did not prepare accordingly for the stated criteria.

0 Not applicable.

Criteria	Peer	Self	Instructor	Comment
Maxillary Placement				
1. Instructed the patient to turn his or her head toward the assistant with chin raised.				
2. Used cotton pliers to transfer cotton rolls to the mouth.				
3. Positioned the cotton rolls securely in the mucobuccal fold.				
4. Positioned the cotton rolls close to the working field.				
Mandibular Placement				
1. Instructed the patient to turn his or her head toward the assistant with chin lowered.				
2. Used cotton pliers to transfer cotton rolls to the mouth.				
3. Positioned the cotton rolls securely in the mucobuccal fold.				
4. Positioned the second cotton roll in the floor of the mouth between the working field and the tongue.				
5. Positioned cotton rolls close to the working field.				
Cotton Roll Removal				
1. If cotton rolls were dry, moistened them with water from the air-water syringe.				
2. Removed cotton rolls with cotton pliers.				
3. Performed a limited rinse.				
4. Maintained patient comfort and followed appropriate infection-control measures throughout the procedure.				

Total amount of points earned _____

Grade _____ *Instructor's initials* _____

Preparation, Placement, and Removal of the Dental Dam

Performance Objective

The student will prepare, place, stabilize, and remove the dental dam.

Grading Criteria

3 Student meets most of the criteria without assistance.

2 Student requires assistance to meet the stated criteria.

1 Student did not prepare accordingly for the stated criteria.

0 Not applicable.

Criteria	Peer	Self	Instructor	Comment
Preparing the Dental Dam				
1. Selected correct setup for the procedure.				
2. Used a mouth mirror and explorer to examine the site to be isolated.				
3. Flossed all contacts involved in placement of dental dam.				
4. Correctly punched the dam for the teeth to be isolated.				
5. Selected the correct size of clamp and tied a ligature to it.				
6. Placed prepared clamp in the dental dam forceps in the position of use.				
Dental Dam Placement				
1. Prepared the dental dam material and clamp for placement.				
2. Seated the clamp so that it is secure around the anchor tooth.				
3. Slid the dam over the clamp, making sure to pull the ligature through the keyhole of the dam.				
4. Positioned the dental dam frame correctly, making sure to fasten all notches to the dam.				
5. Slid the dam through all contacts using floss to push the dam interproximally.				
6. Inverted the dental dam using floss, air, or a blunted instrument.				
7. Ensured that the dam was ligated and stabilized.				

Criteria	Peer	Self	Instructor	Comment
Dental Dam Removal				
1. Removed the stabilization ligature and saliva ejector.				
2. Cut the dental dam septum with scissors.				
3. Removed the dental dam clamp, the dental dam frame, and the used dental dam.				
4. Checked the used dental dam for tears or missing pieces.				
5. Used the air-water syringe and HVE tip to rinse the patient's mouth.				
6. Gently wiped debris from the area around the patient's mouth.				
7. Maintained patient comfort and followed appropriate infection-control measures throughout the procedure.				

Total amount of points earned _____

Grade _____ *Instructor's initials* _____

11 The Dental Patient

TRUE/FALSE

_____ 1. A patient record is commonly referred to as the "patient's plan."

_____ 2. The medical history update form should be completed and signed by the patient at every appointment.

_____ 3. Before a consultation can take place between a physician and dentist, the patient must sign a release of information form.

_____ 4. When taking a pulse reading, it is also important to note any changes in rhythm and depth.

_____ 5. An HIPAA policy should be in place and visible in every dental office.

_____ 6. Vital signs are indicators of a patient's overall health. They include temperature, pulse, weight, and blood pressure.

_____ 7. A patient's temperature is taken with a thermometer.

_____ 8. In a patient with a blood pressure reading of 132/78, the systolic reading would be the lower number.

_____ 9. The instrument used to amplify the blood pumping through an artery is the sphygmomanometer.

_____ 10. The normal respiration rate for children is 10 to 20 breaths per minute.

MATCHING

_____ 11. The patient's past and present physical condition.

_____ 12. A patient's agreement of treatment

_____ 13. Attention to drug sensitivities, allergic reactions, premedications, or precautions

_____ 14. Indication for a change in a medical history

_____ 15. Treatment plan in a sequenced format

A. Dental problem list

B. Medical alert

C. Medical history update

D. Informed consent

E. Medical history

SHORT ANSWER

16. List three reasons why it is important to have an updated medical history for every patient.

17. Describe the three most common locations to detect a patient's pulse and how these sites are normally used.

18. What is the normal sequence when taking a patient's vital signs?

19. List some of the most common allergies that a patient may have that would be noted in the patient record.

20. You are taking a blood pressure on a new patient. Because you do not have a previous reading, how do you know how high to pump the sphygmomanometer?

Registering a New Patient

Performance Objective

The student will use the appropriate forms to gather patient registration and medical history information.

Grading Criteria

3 Student meets most of the criteria without assistance.

2 Student requires assistance to meet the stated criteria.

1 Student did not prepare accordingly for the stated criteria.

0 Not applicable.

Criteria	Peer	Self	Instructor	Comment
1. Explained the need for the form to be completed.				
2. Provided the patient with a pen and form on a clipboard.				
3. Offered assistance to the patient in completing the form.				
4. Reviewed the completed form to determine if there were questions that were not answered.				
5. Reviewed the completed form for necessary information.				
6. Asked questions that required clarification.				
7. In a private setting, such as the treatment room, asked the patient about information that was not clear.				
8. Verified the patient's signature and date on the form.				

Total amount of points earned _____

Grade _____ *Instructor's initials* _____

Performance Objective

To obtain a completed medical and dental health history.

Grading Criteria

3 Student meets most of the criteria without assistance.

2 Student requires assistance to meet the stated criteria.

1 Student did not prepare accordingly for the stated criteria.

0 Not applicable.

Criteria	Peer	Self	Instructor	Comment
1. Explained the need for the form to be completed.				
2. Provided the patient with a pen and form on a clipboard.				
3. Offered assistance to the patient in completing the form.				
4. Reviewed the completed form for necessary information.				
5. Asked questions that required clarification.				
6. Verified the patient's signature and date on the form.				

Total amount of points earned _____

Grade _____ *Instructor's initials* _____

Taking an Oral Temperature Reading With a Digital Thermometer

Performance Objective

The student will obtain and record an oral temperature.

Grading Criteria

3 Student meets most of the criteria without assistance.

2 Student requires assistance to meet the stated criteria.

1 Student did not prepare accordingly for the stated criteria.

0 Not applicable.

Criteria	Peer	Self	Instructor	Comment
1. Obtained the equipment and supplies required for taking an oral temperature.				
2. Placed on personal protective equipment.				
3. Placed a sheath over the probe of the digital thermometer.				
4. Turned the thermometer on and gently placed it under the patient's tongue.				
5. Left the thermometer in place for the appropriate time, then removed it from the patient's mouth.				
6. Reviewed the temperature reading and recorded it in the patient record.				
7. Turned the thermometer off, removed and disposed of the sheath, and disinfected the thermometer as recommended.				

Total amount of points earned _____

Grade _____ *Instructor's initials* _____

Performance Objective

The student will take and record a patient's pulse.

Grading Criteria

3 Student meets most of the criteria without assistance.

2 Student requires assistance to meet the stated criteria.

1 Student did not prepare accordingly for the stated criteria.

0 Not applicable.

Criteria	Peer	Self	Instructor	Comment
1. Obtained the equipment and supplies required for taking a pulse.				
2. Placed on personal protective equipment.				
3. Seated the patient in an upright position.				
4. Placed the tips of index and middle fingers on the patient's radial artery.				
5. Felt for the patient's pulse before counting.				
6. Counted the pulse for 30 seconds and multiplied by 2 for a 1-minute reading.				
7. Recorded the rate along with any distinct changes in rhythm.				

Total amount of points earned _____

Grade _____ *Instructor's initials* _____

Taking a Patient's Respiration

Performance Objective

The student will obtain and record a patient's respiration.

Grading Criteria

3 Student meets most of the criteria without assistance.

2 Student requires assistance to meet the stated criteria.

1 Student did not prepare accordingly for the stated criteria.

0 Not applicable.

Criteria	Peer	Self	Instructor	Comment
1. Obtained the equipment and supplies required for taking a respiration.				
2. Placed on personal protective equipment.				
3. Seated the patient and maintained position as in taking the pulse.				
4. Counted the rise and fall of the patient's chest for 30 seconds.				
5. Multiplied the count by 2 for a 1-minute reading.				
6. Recorded the rate in the patient's record.				

Total amount of points earned _____

Grade _____ *Instructor's initials* _____

Taking a Patient's Blood Pressure

Performance Objective

The student will obtain and record a patient's blood pressure.

Grading Criteria

3 Student meets most of the criteria without assistance.

2 Student requires assistance to meet the stated criteria.

1 Student did not prepare accordingly for the stated criteria.

0 Not applicable.

Criteria	Peer	Self	Instructor	Comment
1. Obtained the equipment and supplies required for taking a blood pressure.				
2. Placed on personal protective equipment.				
3. Had patient seated with the arm extended at heart level and supported.				
4. Rolled up the patient's sleeve if possible.				
5. Palpated the patient's brachial artery to feel for a pulse.				
6. Counted the patient's brachial pulse for 30 seconds.				
7. Multiplied the count by 2 for a 1-minute reading.				
8. Added 40 mm Hg to get inflation level.				
9. Readied the cuff by expelling any air.				
10. Placed the cuff around the patient's arm 1 inch above antecubital space, with arrow over the brachial artery.				
11. Tightened the cuff and closed it using the Velcro tabs.				
12. Placed earpieces of stethoscope properly.				
13. Placed stethoscope disk over site of brachial artery.				
14. Grasped rubber bulb, lock valve, and inflated cuff to note reading.				
15. Slowly released the valve and listened for sounds.				
16. Slowly continued to release air from the cuff until the last sound was heard.				
17. Recorded a reading and indicated which arm was used.				
18. Disinfected the stethoscope.				

Total amount of points earned _____

Grade _____ *Instructor's initials* _____

12 The Dental Examination

TRUE/FALSE

_____ 1. The identification of a disease is called a diagnosis.

_____ 2. Dental charting can be described by the dental team as "shorthand."

_____ 3. In an anatomic charting diagram, the illustration of each tooth resembles circles divided into segments.

_____ 4. When charting, blue or black represents dental treatment that has to be completed.

_____ 5. The charting abbreviation for mesial-occlusal-distal-lingual is MODL.

_____ 6. Intraoral imaging provides a visual evaluation of bone and tissue that cannot be seen by other means.

_____ 7. Study casts are considered as a component of the dental examination.

_____ 8. To feel or touch something is palpation.

_____ 9. A thorough oral examination includes a careful examination of the neck, face, lips, and all of the soft tissues in the mouth.

_____ 10. It is common practice for the dental assistant to perform the periodontal examination for a patient.

MATCHING

_____ 11. Decay in pits and fissures on the occlusal surfaces of teeth

_____ 12. Decay, abrasion, or defects on the incisal edge of anterior teeth and occlusal surfaces of posterior teeth

_____ 13. Decay on proximal surfaces of incisors and canines

_____ 14. Smooth surface decay occurring on the gingival third of the facial or lingual surfaces

_____ 15. Decay on the proximal surfaces of premolars and molars involving two or more surfaces

_____ 16. Decay on the proximal surfaces of incisors and canines also involving the incisal angle

A. Class III

B. Class I

C. Class VI

D. Class II

E. Class IV

F. Class V

17. Describe the three types of treatment plans that may be prescribed for a patient, depending on need.

18. Fill in the condition to describe each of the charting symbols below.

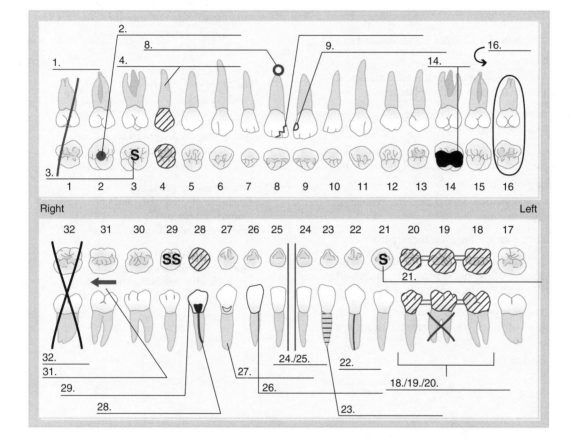

Performance Objective

The student will demonstrate the proper technique for performing a soft-tissue examination.

Grading Criteria

3 Student meets most of the criteria without assistance.

2 Student requires assistance to meet the stated criteria.

1 Student did not prepare accordingly for the stated criteria.

0 Not applicable.

Criteria	Peer	Self	Instructor	Comment
1. Obtained the equipment and supplies required for the procedure.				
2. Escorted the patient to the treatment area, observing the patient's general appearance, speech, and behavior.				
3. Placed on personal protective equipment.				
4. Seated the patient in the dental chair in an upright position.				
5. Explained the procedure to the patient.				
Extraoral Features				
1. Examined the patient's face, neck, and ears for asymmetry or abnormal swelling.				
2. Looked for abnormal tissue changes, skin abrasions, and discolorations.				
3. Evaluated the texture, color, and continuity of the vermilion border, commissures of the lips, philtrum, and smile line.				
4. Documented findings in the patient record.				
Cervical Lymph Nodes				
1. Positioned self in front and to the side of the patient.				
2. Examined the right side of the neck using the fingers and thumb of the right hand to follow the chain of lymph nodes starting in front of the ear and continuing to the collarbone.				
3. Examined the left side of the neck in the same manner.				
4. Documented all findings in the patient record.				

Criteria	Peer	Self	Instructor	Comment
Temporomandibular Joint (TMJ)				
1. Evaluated TMJ movement in centric, lateral, protrusive, and retrusive movements. Asked the patient to open and close the mouth normally and move the jaw from side to side.				
2. Listened for noise in the TMJ as the patient opened and closed the mouth.				
3. Noted in patient record any abnormalities.				
Indications of Oral Habits				
1. Looked for oral habits of thumb sucking, tongue-thrust swallow, mouth breathing, and tobacco use.				
2. Looked for signs of oral habits, such as bruxism, grinding, and clenching.				
Interior of the Lips				
1. Examined the mucosa and labial frenum of the patient's upper lip.				
2. Examined the mucosa and labial frenum of the patient's lower lip.				
3. Palpated tissues to detect lumps or abnormalities.				
Oral Mucosa and Tongue				
1. Palpated the tissue of the buccal mucosa.				
2. Examined the tissue covering the hard palate.				
3. Examined the buccal mucosa and the opening of Stensen's duct.				
4. Evaluated the patient's tongue by pulling it forward and side to side, noting color, papillae, and abnormalities.				
5. Examined the uvula and the base of the tongue.				
Floor of the Mouth				
6. Palpated the soft tissues of the face above and below the mandible.				
7. Palpated the interior of the floor of the mouth.				
8. Observed the quantity and consistency of the flow of the saliva.				
9. Documented all information accurately in the patient record.				

Total amount of points earned _____

Grade _____ Instructor's initials _____

Charting of Teeth

Performance Objective

When provided with a patient chart and colored pencils, the student will demonstrate the proper technique for recording the dentist's findings as dictated during an examination.

Grading Criteria

3 Student meets most of the criteria without assistance.

2 Student requires assistance to meet the stated criteria.

1 Student did not prepare accordingly for the stated criteria.

0 Not applicable.

Criteria	Peer	Self	Instructor	Comment
1. Obtained the equipment and supplies required for the procedure.				
2. Seated the patient in the dental chair in a supine position and draped with a patient napkin.				
3. Had colored pencils, eraser, and clinical examination form readily available.				
4. Recorded specific notations the operator called out for each tooth.				
5. Throughout the procedure used the air syringe to clean the mouth mirror.				
6. Adjusted the operating light as necessary.				
7. Accurately read back the operator's findings.				

Total amount of points earned _____

Grade _____ *Instructor's initials* _____

Recording the Completed Dental Treatment

Performance Objective

The student will record dental treatment and services accurately, completely, and legibly.

Grading Criteria

3 Student meets most of the criteria without assistance.

2 Student requires assistance to meet the stated criteria.

1 Student did not prepare accordingly for the stated criteria.

0 Not applicable.

Criteria	Peer	Self	Instructor	Comment
1. Made all entries in black ink.				
2. Ensured that entries were legible.				
3. Ensured that entries were made in the proper sequence.				
4. Provided correct tooth numbers.				
5. Provided correct tooth surfaces.				
6. Accurately recorded all treatment entries.				
7. Accurately read back the entries.				

Total amount of points earned _____

Grade _____ *Instructor's initials* _____

13 Medical Emergencies in the Dental Office

TRUE/FALSE

_____ 1. The best way to help prevent a potential medical emergency is to have a complete and updated medical history.

_____ 2. The standard of care for an emergency procedure requires that the dental team be competent in CPR and the administration of life-saving drugs.

_____ 3. A list of emergency phone numbers should be noted in every patient record.

_____ 4. Oxygen is the most frequently used drug in a medical emergency.

_____ 5. The diagnosis of a specific medical emergency is the responsibility of everyone on the dental team.

_____ 6. The business staff would be most likely to call for emergency service and then remain on the phone.

_____ 7. Epinephrine would be the drug of choice in the emergency kit for an acute allergic reaction.

_____ 8. A patient with a history of angina would commonly carry Albuterol with them for chest pain.

_____ 9. A sign is what you observe in the patient.

_____ 10. In most areas, the emergency medical service (EMS) can be reached at 919.

MATCHING

_____ 11. Sudden coughing, clutching the throat

_____ 12. Localized itching

_____ 13. Abnormal increase in blood glucose

_____ 14. Wheezing with narrowing airway

_____ 15. Patient placed in upright position too fast

_____ 16. Severe chest pain

_____ 17. Rapid shallow breathing

_____ 18. Interruption of blood flow to the brain

_____ 19. Commonly known as fainting

_____ 20. Neurologic disorder

_____ 21. Heart attack

A. Syncope

B. Postural hypotension

C. Hyperventilation

D. Airway obstruction

E. Asthma

F. Allergic reaction

G. Angina

H. Myocardial infarction

I. Hyperglycemia

J. Cerebrovascular

K. Seizure

22. List the commonly assigned responsibilities of the following members of the dental team in an emergency situation:

    a. Business assistant _____

    _____

    b. Clinical assistant and/or dental hygienist

    _____

    _____

    c. Dentist (clinical assistant or dental hygienist)

    _____

    _____

    d. Other team members

    _____

    _____

23. Describe the difference between a symptom and a sign.

Performing Cardiopulmonary Resuscitation

Performance Objective

The student will use an American Heart Association–approved mannequin to demonstrate the proper technique for performing cardiopulmonary resuscitation (CPR).

Grading Criteria

3 Student meets most of the criteria without assistance.

2 Student requires assistance to meet the stated criteria.

1 Student did not prepare accordingly for the stated criteria.

0 Not applicable.

Criteria	Peer	Self	Instructor	Comment
1. Approached victim and checked for signs of breathing, coughing, or movement.				
2. Asked "Are you OK?"				
3. If no response, called for assistance and for someone to call 911.				
4. Tilted the victim's head and lifted the chin. Looked, listened, and felt for signs of breathing and pulse. Technique should include placing the ear over the mouth, watching the chest rise and fall, and feeling the carotid artery for a pulse.				
5. If no signs of breathing, placed a CPR mouth barrier over the mouth and began rescue breathing. Technique should include pinching the nose tightly with thumb and forefinger.				
6. Gave two full breaths.				
7. If no signs of pulse, knelt at victim's side, opposite chest, and placed heel of hand on victim's chest with other hand on top.				
8. Gave 15 compressions 1½ to 2 inches in depth. Did not remove hands from location.				
9. Completed four cycles of 2:15 chest compressions and breaths.				
10. Reassessed victim.				
11. Continued until medical service arrived.				

Total amount of points earned _____

Grade _____ *Instructor's initials* _____

Responding to the Patient With an Obstructed Airway

Performance Objective

The student will demonstrate the proper technique for the Heimlich maneuver.

Grading Criteria

3 Student meets most of the criteria without assistance.

2 Student requires assistance to meet the stated criteria.

1 Student did not prepare accordingly for the stated criteria.

0 Not applicable.

Criteria	Peer	Self	Instructor	Comment
1. If the victim could not speak, cough, or breathe, immediately called for assistance.				
2. Made a fist and placed the thumb side of the hand against the victim's abdomen just above the belly button.				
3. Grasped the fist with the other hand and forcefully thrusted both hands with an inward and upward motion.				
4. Repeated thrusts until object was expelled.				

Total amount of points earned _____

Grade _____ *Instructor's initials* _____

Performance Objective

The student will act out and verbally respond to an unconscious patient.

Grading Criteria

3 Student meets most of the criteria without assistance.

2 Student requires assistance to meet the stated criteria.

1 Student did not prepare accordingly for the stated criteria.

0 Not applicable.

Criteria	Peer	Self	Instructor	Comment
1. Placed the patient in subsupine position with head lower than feet.				
2. Called for assistance.				
3. Loosened any binding clothing.				
4. Had an ammonia inhalant ready to administer under the patient's nose.				
5. Had oxygen ready for use.				
6. Monitored and recorded vital signs.				

Total amount of points earned _____

Grade _____ *Instructor's initials* _____

Responding to the Patient With a Breathing Problem

Performance Objective

The student will act out and verbally respond to a patient with a breathing problem.

Grading Criteria

3 Student meets most of the criteria without assistance.

2 Student requires assistance to meet the stated criteria.

1 Student did not prepare accordingly for the stated criteria.

0 Not applicable.

Criteria	Peer	Self	Instructor	Comment
1. Called for medical assistance.				
2. Placed the patient in a comfortable position.				
3. Used a quiet voice to calm and reassure the patient.				
4. If asthma induced, had the patient self-medicate with inhaler.				
5. If hyperventilating, had a paper bag ready for the patient to breathe into.				
6. Administered oxygen if needed.				
7. Monitored and recorded vital signs.				

Total amount of points earned _____

Grade _____ *Instructor's initials* _____

Responding to the Patient Experiencing a Convulsive Seizure

Performance Objective

The student will act out and verbally respond to a patient experiencing a convulsive seizure.

Grading Criteria

3 Student meets most of the criteria without assistance.

2 Student requires assistance to meet the stated criteria.

1 Student did not prepare accordingly for the stated criteria.

0 Not applicable.

Criteria	Peer	Self	Instructor	Comment
1. Called for medical assistance.				
2. Placed the patient in a comfortable position, preferably flat on the floor.				
3. Prevented self-injury of the patient during the seizure.				
4. Readied the anticonvulsant from the drug kit if needed.				
5. Initiated basic life support if needed.				
6. Monitored and recorded vital signs.				

Total amount of points earned _____

Grade _____ *Instructor's initials* _____

Responding to the Patient Experiencing a Diabetic Emergency

Performance Objective

The student will act out and verbally respond to a patient experiencing a diabetic emergency.

Grading Criteria

3 Student meets most of the criteria without assistance.

2 Student requires assistance to meet the stated criteria.

1 Student did not prepare accordingly for the stated criteria.

0 Not applicable.

Criteria	Peer	Self	Instructor	Comment
1. Called for medical assistance.				
2. If the patient was conscious, asked questions regarding when insulin was last taken.				
3. Retrieved the patient's insulin if hyperglycemic or gave concentrated carbohydrate if hypoglycemic.				
4. If the patient was unconscious, provided basic life support.				
5. Monitored and recorded vital signs.				

Total amount of points earned _____

Grade _____ *Instructor's initials* _____

Responding to the Patient With Chest Pain

Performance Objective

The student will act out and verbally respond to a patient with chest pain.

Grading Criteria

3 Student meets most of the criteria without assistance.

2 Student requires assistance to meet the stated criteria.

1 Student did not prepare accordingly for the stated criteria.

0 Not applicable.

Criteria	Peer	Self	Instructor	Comment
1. Called for medical assistance.				
2. Placed the patient in an upright position.				
3. Obtained nitroglycerin from the patient or emergency kit.				
4. Administered oxygen.				
5. Monitored and recorded vital signs.				

Total amount of points earned _____

Grade _____ *Instructor's initials* _____

Responding to the Patient Experiencing a Stroke (CVA)

Performance Objective

The student will act out and verbally respond to a patient experiencing a stroke (cerebral vascular accident [CVA]).

Grading Criteria

3 Student meets most of the criteria without assistance.

2 Student requires assistance to meet the stated criteria.

1 Student did not prepare accordingly for the stated criteria.

0 Not applicable.

Criteria	Peer	Self	Instructor	Comment
1. Called for medical assistance.				
2. Initiated basic life support if the patient was unconscious.				
3. Monitored and recorded vital signs.				

Total amount of points earned _____

Grade _____ *Instructor's initials* _____

Responding to the Patient Experiencing an Allergic Reaction

Performance Objective

The student will act out and verbally respond to a patient experiencing an allergic reaction.

Grading Criteria

3 Student meets most of the criteria without assistance.

2 Student requires assistance to meet the stated criteria.

1 Student did not prepare accordingly for the stated criteria.

0 Not applicable.

Criteria	Peer	Self	Instructor	Comment
1. Called for medical assistance.				
2. Readied an antihistamine or epinephrine for administration if needed.				
3. Initiated basic life support if needed.				
4. Referred the patient for medical consultation.				
5. Monitored and recorded vital signs.				

Total amount of points earned _____

Grade _____ *Instructor's initials* _____

14 Pain and Anxiety Control

TRUE/FALSE

_____ 1. A vasoconstrictor can be added to a local anesthetic to cause a blood vessel to constrict.

_____ 2. The anesthetic cartridge is also referred to as the syringe.

_____ 3. A patient with a cold could have a condition that would make nitrous oxide/oxygen a contraindication for treatment.

_____ 4. The color coding system designed for local anesthetic is blue and green.

_____ 5. Duration is the time frame from when an injection is given until the numbing sensation is gone.

_____ 6. Topical anesthetic provides a temporary numbing effect on the nerve endings on the surface of the oral mucosa.

_____ 7. Block anesthesia involves injecting the anesthetic solution into the tissues near the apices of the tooth to be treated.

_____ 8. The transfer of a syringe should take place in the operator's zone.

_____ 9. Analgesics are drugs that dull the perception of pain without producing unconsciousness.

_____ 10. Tylenol is a brand name of acetaminophen.

MATCHING

Match the type of drug with its drug category.

_____ 11. Penicillin   A. Analgesic

_____ 12. Ibuprofen   B. Antibiotic

_____ 13. Morphine   C. Sedative

_____ 14. Valium   D. Narcotic

Match the following parts of the anesthetic syringe.

_____ 15. Thumb ring

_____ 16. Harpoon

_____ 17. Barrel of syringe

_____ 18. Finger grip

_____ 19. Piston rod

_____ 20. Threaded tip

A. Hub where the needle is screwed onto the syringe

B. Where the dentist holds the syringe firmly

C. Sharp hooklike component that fits into the rubber stopper of the cartridge

D. Holds the anesthetic cartridge

E. C-shaped portion of the area grasped by the operator

F. Pushes down the rubber stopper on the anesthetic cartridge

SHORT ANSWER

21. List five specific health conditions that would impact the selection of local anesthetics.

22. List three advantages of using nitrous oxide analgesia.

127

Applying a Topical Anesthetic

Performance Objective

The student will select the necessary setup, identify the injection site, and apply topical anesthetic.

Grading Criteria

3 Student meets most of the criteria without assistance.

2 Student requires assistance to meet the stated criteria.

1 Student did not prepare accordingly for the stated criteria.

0 Not applicable.

Criteria	Peer	Self	Instructor	Comment
Preparation				
1. Gathered the appropriate setup.				
2. Used a sterile cotton-tipped applicator to remove a small amount of topical anesthetic ointment from the container; replaced the cover immediately.				
3. Explained the procedure to the patient.				
4. Determined the injection site.				
5. Wiped the injection site dry using a sterile 2-by-2-inch gauze pad.				
Placement				
1. Applied topical anesthetic ointment to the injection site only.				
2. Left the topical anesthetic ointment in contact with the oral tissues for 2 to 5 minutes.				
3. Removed the cotton-tipped applicator just before the injection was made by the dentist.				
4. Maintained patient comfort and followed appropriate infection-control measures throughout the procedure.				

Total amount of points earned _____

Grade _____ *Instructor's initials* _____

Assisting in the Assembly and Administration of Local Anesthesia

Performance Objective

The student will select the necessary setup, prepare an aspirating type of syringe for local anesthetic injection, and assist in the administration.

Grading Criteria

3 Student meets most of the criteria without assistance.

2 Student requires assistance to meet the stated criteria.

1 Student did not prepare accordingly for the stated criteria.

0 Not applicable.

Criteria	Peer	Self	Instructor	Comment
1. Gathered the necessary instruments and supplies.				
2. Inspected the syringe, needle, and anesthetic cartridge, and then prepared the syringe out of the patient's sight.				
3. Double-checked the anesthetic cartridge to confirm that the anesthetic is the type the dentist indicated.				
Inserting the Cartridge				
1. Retracted the piston using the thumb ring and then inserted the anesthetic cartridge with the rubber stopper end first.				
2. Released the piston and gently engaged the harpoon.				
3. Gently pulled back on the thumb ring to be certain the harpoon was securely in place.				
Attaching the Needle				
1. Removed the plastic cap from the syringe end of the needle and screwed the needle onto the syringe.				
2. Loosened the colored plastic cap from the injection end of the needle.				
Transferring the Syringe				
1. Transferred the syringe below the patient's chin or behind the patient's head as instructed.				
2. Took appropriate safety precaution measures while transferring the syringe.				

Criteria	Peer	Self	Instructor	Comment
Disassembling the Used Syringe				
1. Retracted the piston of the syringe by pulling back on the thumb ring.				
2. While still retracting the piston, removed the anesthetic cartridge from the syringe.				
3. Unscrewed and removed the needle from the syringe.				
4. Disposed of the needle in an appropriate sharps container.				
5. Disposed of the used cartridge in the appropriate waste container.				
6. Followed appropriate infection-control measures throughout the procedure.				

Total amount of points earned _____

Grade _____ *Instructor's initials* _____

Assisting in the Administration and Monitoring of Nitrous Oxide/Oxygen Sedation (Expanded Function)

Performance Objective

The student will assist with the administration of nitrous oxide analgesia by monitoring the patient's reactions and recording appropriate information in the patient's record.

Grading Criteria

3 Student meets most of the criteria without assistance.

2 Student requires assistance to meet the stated criteria.

1 Student did not prepare accordingly for the stated criteria.

0 Not applicable.

Criteria	Peer	Self	Instructor	Comment
Before Administration				
1. Checked the nitrous oxide and oxygen tanks for adequate supply.				
2. Gathered appropriate supplies and placed a sterile mask of the appropriate size on the tubing.				
3. Updated the patient's health history, then took and recorded the patient's blood pressure and pulse.				
4. Familiarized the patient with the experience of nitrous oxide analgesia.				
5. Placed the patient in a supine position.				
6. Assisted the patient with placement of the mask.				
7. Made necessary adjustments to the mask and tubing to ensure proper fit.				
During Administration				
1. At the dentist's direction, adjusted the flow of oxygen to the established tidal volume.				
2. At the dentist's direction, adjusted the flow of nitrous oxide and oxygen.				
3. Noted on the patient's chart the time and volumes of gas needed to achieve baseline.				
4. Monitored the patient throughout the procedure.				

Criteria	Peer	Self	Instructor	Comment
Oxygenation				
1. At the dentist's direction, turned off the flow of nitrous oxide and increased the flow of oxygen.				
2. After oxygenation was complete, removed the nosepiece, and then slowly returned the patient to the upright position.				
3. Recorded on the patient's record the concentrations of gases administered and any unusual patient reactions to the analgesia.				
4. Maintained patient comfort and followed appropriate infection-control measures throughout the procedure.				

Total amount of points earned _____

Grade _____ *Instructor's initials* _____

15 Radiation Safety and Production of X-Rays

TRUE/FALSE

_____ 1. When x-rays strike patients' tissues, ionization results.

_____ 2. The amount of radiation that is absorbed by the tissues is called dose equivalence.

_____ 3. The maximum permissible dose (MPD) for occupationally exposed persons is 5.0 rem.

_____ 4. The fastest speed film used in dentistry is F speed.

_____ 5. Collimation is used to remove the longer low-energy x-rays from the x-ray beam.

FILL IN THE BLANK

6. _____ is when small amounts of radiation are absorbed over a long period of time.

7. _____ is when large amounts of radiation are absorbed in a short time.

8. _____ effects of radiation are those that build up over a lifetime.

9. _____ is used to restrict the size and shape of the x-ray beam.

10. _____ removes the longer wavelength, low-energy rays from the beam.

MULTIPLE CHOICE

11. When should the dental assistant hold the film in the patient's mouth during exposure?
    a. for young children
    b. for patients with disabilities
    c. for edentulous patients when the exposure time is less
    d. never

12. Images appearing dark or black on the radiograph are termed:
    a. radiolucent
    b. low contrast
    c. radiopaque
    d. distorted

13. Distortion of the image can be caused by:
    a. object-film distance
    b. source-film distance
    c. movement
    d. all of the above

14. The milliamperage selector controls:
    a. the number of electrons that are produced
    b. the penetrating power
    c. the quality of the x-ray
    d. all of the above

15. The exposure time is measured in units of:
    a. fractions of a second called impulses
    b. seconds
    c. minutes
    d. all of the above

Label the parts of a dental x-ray tube.

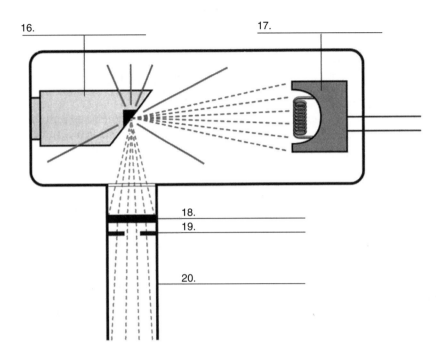

16 Oral Radiography

TRUE/FALSE

_____ 1. The bisection of the angle technique is preferred because it is more accurate.

_____ 2. When using the paralleling technique, the jaw being radiographed is adjusted parallel to the floor when the film packet is in position.

_____ 3. The periapical radiograph is the most accurate for diagnosing dental decay.

_____ 4. Incorrect horizontal angulation is responsible for closed contacts on the radiograph.

_____ 5. When the vertical angulation is too flat (low), the image will be foreshortened.

SHORT ANSWER

List the steps in processing radiographs.

6.

7.

8.

9.

10.

FILL IN THE BLANK

11. _____ films are caused by overdevelopment.

12. _____ films are caused by underdevelopment.

13. _____ films are caused by improper safelight, expired film, or stray radiation.

14. _____ on the film are caused by fingers wet from water and/or chemicals.

15. _____ on the film can be caused by fingernails or clips.

MULTIPLE CHOICE

16. After the film has been exposed, the invisible image on the film is called the:
    a. lead foil
    b. latent image
    c. radiolucent image
    d. radiopaque image

17. How many sizes of dental film are commonly used?
    a. 2
    b. 3
    c. 4
    d. 5

18. Which of the following are common sources of disease transmission during radiography?
    a. x-ray machine arm, head, and position indicating device
    b. control panel and exposure button
    c. lead apron
    d. all of the above

19. Dental film should be stored in a way to protect them from:
    a. light and heat
    b. scatter radiation
    c. chemicals
    d. all of the above

20. Which of the following infection-control measures are **not** used in dental radiography?
    a. PPE (personal protective equipment)
    b. sterilization of film packets
    c. surface barriers
    d. standard operating procedures

Identify the types of dental radiographs.

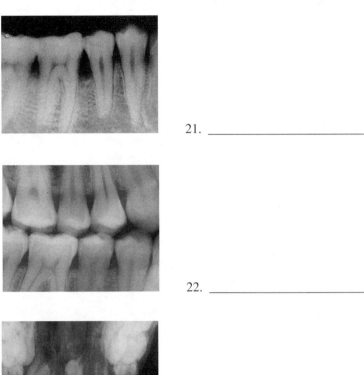

21. _____

22. _____

23. _____

Practicing Infection Control During Film Exposure

Performance Objective

The student will demonstrate the proper technique for implementing appropriate infection-control procedures during film exposure.

Grading Criteria

3 Student meets most of the criteria without assistance.

2 Student requires assistance to meet the stated criteria.

1 Student did not prepare accordingly for the stated criteria.

0 Not applicable.

Criteria	Peer	Self	Instructor	Comment
1. Washed and dried hands and placed barriers.				
2. Washed and dried hands and put on gloves.				
3. Wiped the exposed packet on the paper towel.				
4. When finished exposing films and while still gloved, discarded the paper towel.				
5. Removed gloves and washed hands before leaving the treatment room.				
6. Carried the cup or bag of exposed films to the processing area.				

Total amount of points earned _____

Grade _____ *Instructor's initials* _____

Performance Objective

The student will demonstrate the proper technique for assembling a localizer-ring film-holding instrument.

Grading Criteria

3 Student meets most of the criteria without assistance.

2 Student requires assistance to meet the stated criteria.

1 Student did not prepare accordingly for the stated criteria.

0 Not applicable.

Criteria	Peer	Self	Instructor	Comment
1. Assembled the instruments for the area to be radiographed.				
2. Placed the film into the backing plate.				
3. Used the entire horizontal length of the bite-block.				
4. Placed the anterior edge of the bite-block on the incisal or occlusal surfaces of the teeth being radiographed.				
5. Instructed the patient to close slowly but firmly.				
6. Placed a cotton roll between the bite-block and the teeth of the opposite arch.				
7. Moved the localizer ring down the indicator rod into position.				
8. Aligned the position-indicator device (PID).				
9. Exposed the film, then removed the film and holding device from the patient's mouth.				

Total amount of points earned _____

Grade _____ *Instructor's initials* _____

Producing a Full-Mouth Radiographic Survey Using the Paralleling Technique

Performance Objective

The student will produce a full-mouth radiographic survey using the proper paralleling technique.

Grading Criteria

3 Student meets most of the criteria without assistance.

2 Student requires assistance to meet the stated criteria.

1 Student did not prepare accordingly for the stated criteria.

0 Not applicable.

Criteria	Peer	Self	Instructor	Comment
Preparation				
1. Determined the number and type of films to be exposed.				
2. Labeled a paper cup or plastic bag and placed it outside of the room where the x-ray machine is used.				
3. Turned on the x-ray machine and checked the basic settings.				
4. Washed hands.				
5. Dispensed the desired number of films and stored them outside of the room where the x-ray machine is used.				
6. Placed all necessary barriers.				
Positioning the Patient				
1. Adjusted the chair with the patient positioned upright. Adjusted the level of the chair to a comfortable working height for the operator.				
2. Adjusted the headrest to support and position the patient's head so that the upper arch is parallel to the floor and the midsagittal (midline) plane is perpendicular to the floor.				
3. Asked the patient to remove eyeglasses and bulky earrings.				
4. Draped the patient with a lead apron and thyroid collar.				
5. Washed hands and put on clean exam gloves.				
6. Asked the patient to remove any removable prosthetic appliances from his or her mouth.				
7. Opened the package and assembled the sterile film-holding instruments.				
8. Used a mouth mirror to inspect the oral cavity.				

145

Criteria	Peer	Self	Instructor	Comment
Maxillary Central/Lateral Incisor Region				
1. Inserted the film packet vertically into the anterior block.				
2. Positioned the film.				
3. Instructed the patient to close slowly but firmly.				
4. Positioned the localizing ring and PID and then exposed the film.				
Maxillary Canine Region				
1. Inserted the film packet vertically into the anterior bite-block.				
2. Positioned the film packet with the canine and first premolar centered.				
3. Instructed the patient to close slowly but firmly.				
4. Positioned the localizing ring and PID and then exposed the film.				
Maxillary Premolar Region				
1. Inserted the film packet horizontally into the posterior bite-block.				
2. Centered the film packet on the second premolar.				
3. With the instrument and film in place, instructed the patient to close slowly but firmly.				
4. Positioned the localizing ring and PID and then exposed the film.				
Maxillary Molar Region				
1. Inserted the film packet horizontally into the posterior bite-block.				
2. Centered the film packet on the second molar.				
3. With the instrument and film in place, instructed the patient to close slowly but firmly.				
4. Positioned the localizing ring and PID and then exposed the film (as above).				
Mandibular Incisor Region				
1. Inserted the film packet vertically into the anterior bite-block.				
2. Centered the film packet between the central incisors.				
3. With the instrument and film in place, instructed the patient to close slowly but firmly.				
4. Positioned the localizing ring and PID and then exposed the film.				

Criteria	Peer	Self	Instructor	Comment
Mandibular Canine Region				
1. Inserted the film packet vertically into the anterior bite-block.				
2. Centered the film on the canine.				
3. Used a cotton roll between the maxillary teeth and bite-block, if necessary.				
4. With the instrument and film in place, instructed the patient to close slowly but firmly.				
5. Positioned the localizing ring and PID and then exposed the film.				
Mandibular Premolar Region				
1. Inserted the film horizontally into the posterior bite-block.				
2. Centered the film on the contact point between the second premolar and first molar.				
3. With the instrument and film in place, instructed the patient to close slowly but firmly.				
4. Positioned the localizing ring and PID and then exposed the film.				
Mandibular Molar Region				
1. Inserted the film horizontally into the posterior bite-block.				
2. Centered the film on the second molar.				
3. With the instrument and film in place, instructed the patient to close slowly but firmly.				
4. Positioned the localizing ring and PID and then exposed the film.				

Total amount of points earned _____

Grade _____ *Instructor's initials* _____

Producing a Four-Film Radiographic Survey Using the Bite-Wing Technique

Performance Objective

The student will produce a full-mouth radiographic survey using the proper bite-wing technique.

Grading Criteria

3 Student meets most of the criteria without assistance.

2 Student requires assistance to meet the stated criteria.

1 Student did not prepare accordingly for the stated criteria.

0 Not applicable.

Criteria	Peer	Self	Instructor	Comment
1. Placed the film in the patient's mouth for a premolar film.				
2. Placed the film in proper position.				
3. Set the vertical angulation.				
4. Positioned horizontal angulation.				
5. Positioned the PID.				

Total amount of points earned _____

Grade _____ *Instructor's initials* _____

COMPETENCY 16-5

Performance Objective

The student will produce maxillary and mandibular occlusal radiographs using the proper occlusal technique.

Grading Criteria

3 Student meets most of the criteria without assistance.

2 Student requires assistance to meet the stated criteria.

1 Student did not prepare accordingly for the stated criteria.

0 Not applicable.

Criteria	Peer	Self	Instructor	Comment
Maxillary Occlusal Technique				
1. Positioned the patient's head so the film plane was parallel to the floor.				
2. Placed the film packet in the patient's mouth with the white side of the film on the occlusal surfaces of the maxillary teeth.				
3. Placed the film as far posterior as possible.				
4. Positioned the PID so that the central ray was directed at a 65° angle through the bridge of the nose to the center of the film packet.				
5. Pressed the x-ray machine–activating button and made the exposure.				
Mandibular Occlusal Technique				
1. Tilted the patient's head back to a comfortable position, ensuring that the midsagittal plane was vertical.				
2. Placed the film packet in the patient's mouth with the white side of the film on the occlusal surfaces of the mandibular teeth.				
3. Positioned the film as far posterior as possible.				
4. Positioned the PID so that the central ray was directed at 90° (a right angle) to the center of the film packet.				
5. Pressed the x-ray machine–activating button and made the exposure.				

Total amount of points earned _____

Grade _____ *Instructor's initials* _____

Practicing Infection Control in the Darkroom

Performance Objective

The student will demonstrate the proper technique for implementing proper infection control in the darkroom.

Grading Criteria

3 Student meets most of the criteria without assistance.

2 Student requires assistance to meet the stated criteria.

1 Student did not prepare accordingly for the stated criteria.

0 Not applicable.

Criteria	Peer	Self	Instructor	Comment
1. Placed a paper towel and a clean cup on the counter near the processor.				
2. Put on a new pair of gloves.				
3. Opened the film packets and allowed each exposed film to drop onto the paper towel. Ensured that unwrapped films did not come into contact with gloves.				
4. Removed the lead foil from the packet and placed it into the foil container.				
5. Placed the empty film packets into the clean cup.				
6. Discarded the cup and removed gloves with insides turned out and discarded them.				
7. Placed the films into the processor or on developing racks with bare hands.				

Total amount of points earned _____

Grade _____ *Instructor's initials* _____

Practicing Infection Control Using the Daylight Loader

Performance Objective

The student will demonstrate proper infection-control techniques while using the daylight loader.

Grading Criteria

3 Student meets most of the criteria without assistance.

2 Student requires assistance to meet the stated criteria.

1 Student did not prepare accordingly for the stated criteria.

0 Not applicable.

Criteria	Peer	Self	Instructor	Comment
1. Washed and dried hands, then placed a paper towel or piece of plastic as a barrier inside the bottom of the daylight loader.				
2. Placed the cup with the contaminated film, a clean pair of gloves, and a second paper cup on the barrier, and closed the top.				
3. Put clean hands through the sleeves and put on the gloves.				
4. Opened the packets and allowed the films to drop onto the clean barrier, placed the contaminated packets into the second cup, and placed the lead foil into the foil container.				
5. After opening the last packet, removed gloves with insides turned out, and inserted the films into the developing slots.				
6. After inserting the last film, pulled ungloved hands through sleeves.				
7. Opened the top of the loader and carefully pulled the ends of the barrier over the paper cup and used gloves and discarded them. Used care not to touch the contaminated parts of the barrier with bare hands.				
8. Washed and dried hands.				

Total amount of points earned _____

Grade _____ *Instructor's initials* _____

COMPETENCY 16-8

Manual Processing of Dental Radiographs

Performance Objective

The student will demonstrate the proper technique for processing films manually.

Grading Criteria

3 Student meets most of the criteria without assistance.

2 Student requires assistance to meet the stated criteria.

1 Student did not prepare accordingly for the stated criteria.

0 Not applicable.

Criteria	Peer	Self	Instructor	Comment
Preparation Steps				
1. Followed all infection-control steps.				
2. Stirred the solutions and checked solution levels and temperature. The temperature was between 65° F and 70° F.				
3. Labeled the film rack with the patient's name and the date of exposure.				
4. Washed and dried hands and put on gloves.				
5. Turned on the safelight, then turned off the white light.				
6. Opened the film packets and allowed the films to drop onto the clean paper towel. Used care not to touch the films.				
7. Removed contaminated gloves and washed and dried hands.				
Processing Steps				
1. Attached each film to the film rack so that films were parallel and not touching.				
2. Agitated the rack slightly while inserting it into the solution.				
3. Started the timer. The timer was set according to the manufacturer's instructions on the basis of the temperature of the solutions.				
4. Removed the rack of films after the timer went off and rinsed it in running water in the center tank for 20 to 30 seconds.				
5. Determined the fixation time and set the timer. Immersed the rack of films in the fixer tank.				
6. Returned the rack of films to the center tank with circulating water for a minimum of 20 minutes.				
7. Removed the rack of films from the water and allowed it to dry.				
8. When completely dry, removed the films from the rack and mounted them in an appropriately labeled mount.				

Total amount of points earned _____

Grade _____ *Instructor's initials* _____

Processing Dental Radiographs in an Automatic Film Processor

Performance Objective

The student will demonstrate the proper technique for processing dental radiographs in an automatic film processor.

Grading Criteria

3 Student meets most of the criteria without assistance.

2 Student requires assistance to meet the stated criteria.

1 Student did not prepare accordingly for the stated criteria.

0 Not applicable.

Criteria	Peer	Self	Instructor	Comment
1. Before the machine was operational, turned it on and allowed the chemicals to warm up (according to manufacturer's recommendations for proper temperature).				
2. Followed infection-control steps.				
3. Opened film packet. Then removed the black paper and lead foil. Placed the films in the processor.				
4. Fed the films slowly into the machine and kept them straight. Allowed at least 10 seconds between inserting each film into the processor. Alternated slots within the processor when possible.				

Total amount of points earned _____

Grade _____ *Instructor's initials* _____

Mounting Dental Radiographs

Performance Objective

The student will demonstrate the proper technique for mounting a full-mouth series of radiographs.

Grading Criteria

3 Student meets most of the criteria without assistance.

2 Student requires assistance to meet the stated criteria.

1 Student did not prepare accordingly for the stated criteria.

0 Not applicable.

Criteria	Peer	Self	Instructor	Comment
1. Ensured that hands were clean and dry before handling radiographs. Grasped films only at the edges, not on the front or back.				
2. Selected the appropriate-size mount and labeled it with the patient's name and the date the radiographs were exposed.				
3. Arranged the dried radiographs in anatomic order on a piece of clean white paper or on a flat view box.				
4. Once the films were arranged properly, placed them neatly in the mount.				

Total amount of points earned _____

Grade _____ *Instructor's initials* _____

161

Preparing Equipment for Panoramic Radiography

Performance Objective

The student will demonstrate the proper technique for preparing equipment for a panoramic radiograph.

Grading Criteria

3 Student meets most of the criteria without assistance.

2 Student requires assistance to meet the stated criteria.

1 Student did not prepare accordingly for the stated criteria.

0 Not applicable.

Criteria	Peer	Self	Instructor	Comment
1. Loaded the panoramic cassette in the darkroom under safelight conditions. Handled the film only by its edges to prevent fingerprints.				
2. Placed all infection-control barriers and containers.				
3. Covered the bite-block with a disposable plastic barrier. If the bite-block was not covered, sterilized it before using it on the next patient.				
4. Covered or disinfected (or both) any part of the machine that came in contact with the patient.				
5. Set the exposure factors (kilovoltage and milliamperage) according to the manufacturer's recommendations.				
6. Adjusted the machine to accommodate the height of the patient and aligned all movable parts properly.				
7. Loaded the cassette into the carrier of the panoramic unit.				

Total amount of points earned _____

Grade _____ *Instructor's initials* _____

Performance Objective

The student will demonstrate the proper technique for preparing a patient for panoramic radiography.

Grading Criteria

3 Student meets most of the criteria without assistance.

2 Student requires assistance to meet the stated criteria.

1 Student did not prepare accordingly for the stated criteria.

0 Not applicable.

Criteria	Peer	Self	Instructor	Comment
1. Explained the procedure to the patient. Gave the patient the opportunity to ask questions.				
2. Asked the patient to remove all objects from the head and neck area, including eyeglasses, earrings, lip-piercing and tongue-piercing objects, necklaces, napkin chains, hearing aids, hairpins, and complete and partial dentures. Placed objects in separate containers.				
3. Placed a double-sided (for protecting the front and back of the patient) lead apron on the patient or used the style of lead apron recommended by the manufacturer.				

Total amount of points earned _____

Grade _____ *Instructor's initials* _____

Positioning a Patient for Panoramic Radiography

Performance Objective

The student will demonstrate the proper technique for positioning a patient for panoramic radiography.

Grading Criteria

3 Student meets most of the criteria without assistance.

2 Student requires assistance to meet the stated criteria.

1 Student did not prepare accordingly for the stated criteria.

0 Not applicable.

Criteria	Peer	Self	Instructor	Comment
Procedural Steps				
1. Instructed the patient to sit or stand "as tall as possible" with the back straight and erect.				
2. Instructed the patient to bite on the plastic bite-block and slide the upper and lower teeth into the notch (groove) on the end of the bite-block.				
3. Positioned the midsagittal plane perpendicular to the floor.				
4. Positioned the Frankfort plane parallel to the floor.				
5. Instructed the patient to position the tongue on the roof of the mouth and then to close the lips around the bite-block.				
6. After the patient was positioned, instructed the patient to remain still while the machine rotated during exposure.				
7. Exposed the film and proceeded with film processing.				
8. Documented the procedure.				

Total amount of points earned _____

Grade _____ *Instructor's initials* _____

17 Preventive Care

TRUE/FALSE

_____ 1. Fluoridated drinking water contains approximately 1 part per million (ppm) of fluoride.

_____ 2. Fluoride is a naturally occurring mineral.

_____ 3. Flossing is the most effective on occlusal surfaces of the teeth.

_____ 4. Disclosing agents are useful as teaching aids.

_____ 5. An oral health program is based upon motivation and education.

FILL IN THE BLANK

6. _____ can be caused by excessive amounts of fluoride.

7. _____ fluorides are also known as dietary fluorides.

8. _____ fluoride is applied by toothpaste, rinses, and gels.

9. _____ is the process by which decay begins.

10. _____ is the most effective way to learn.

11. A food that is _____ has the ability to cause dental decay.

12. _____ is used to remove plaque from interproximal surfaces.

13. _____ are used to clean large spaces between the teeth.

14. _____ is the process by which decay is stopped.

15. The most commonly recommended method of toothbrushing is the _____ technique.

MULTIPLE CHOICE

16. Which of the following are effective interdental aids?
    a. interproximal brushes
    b. dental floss
    c. rubber and wooden-tip stimulators
    d. all of the above

17. How are systemic fluorides applied?
    a. in toothpaste
    b. in mouth rinses
    c. by drinking fluoridated water
    d. all of the above

18. Which of the following would make a patient high risk for dental decay?
    a. having already had dental decay
    b. living in an area without public water fluoridation
    c. having a limited amount of saliva
    d. all of the above

19. Which of the following foods is the **most** cariogenic?
    a. sweet sticky foods
    b. soft drinks
    c. fruits
    d. vegetables

20. Oral health education **does not** include:
    a. open communication
    b. listening to the patient's concerns
    c. providing reinforcement
    d. lecturing to the patient

Applying Topical Fluoride Gel or Foam

Performance Objective

The student will demonstrate the proper technique for applying a topical fluoride gel or foam.

Grading Criteria

3 Student meets most of the criteria without assistance.

2 Student requires assistance to meet the stated criteria.

1 Student did not prepare accordingly for the stated criteria.

0 Not applicable.

Criteria	Peer	Self	Instructor	Comment
Preparation				
1. Selected the appropriate tray and other materials.				
2. Dispensed the appropriate amount of fluoride material into the tray.				
3. Positioned the patient and provided patient instructions.				
4. Dried the teeth.				
5. Inserted the tray and placed cotton rolls between the arches.				
6. Promptly placed the saliva ejector and tilted the patient's head forward.				
7. Removed the tray without allowing the patient to rinse or swallow.				
8. Used the saliva ejector or HVE tip to remove excess saliva and solution.				
9. Instructed the patient not to rinse, eat, drink, or brush the teeth for at least 30 minutes.				

Total amount of points earned _____

Grade _____ *Instructor's initials* _____

Performance Objective

The student will demonstrate the proper technique for assisting a patient in learning how to use dental floss.

Grading Criteria

3 Student meets most of the criteria without assistance.

2 Student requires assistance to meet the stated criteria.

1 Student did not prepare accordingly for the stated criteria.

0 Not applicable.

Criteria	Peer	Self	Instructor	Comment
1. Dispensed the appropriate amount of dental floss.				
2. Stretched the floss tightly between the fingers and used the thumb and index finger to guide the floss into place.				
3. Held the floss tightly between the thumb and forefinger of each hand.				
4. Passed the floss gently between the teeth.				
5. Curved the floss into a C shape against each tooth and wiped up and down against the tooth surfaces.				
6. Repeated these steps on each side of all teeth in both arches.				
7. Moved a fresh piece of floss into the working position as the floss became frayed or soiled.				
8. Used a bridge threader to floss under any fixed bridges.				

Total amount of points earned _____

Grade _____ *Instructor's initials* _____

18 Coronal Polishing and Dental Sealants

TRUE/FALSE

_____ 1. Placement of dental sealants can be quite painful.

_____ 2. The patient, operator, and assistant must use special protective eyewear when the curing light is in use.

_____ 3. Well-placed dental sealants will last more than 10 years with proper care.

_____ 4. Flossing after a coronal polish will help remove any remaining abrasive agent.

_____ 5. Bristle brushes are recommended for use on exposed cementum or dentin.

FILL IN THE BLANK

6. _____ stains may be removed by scaling or polishing.

7. _____ is a type of sealant material that needs no mixing.

8. A _____ is a finger rest used when performing a coronal polish.

9. A _____ is a procedure in which calculus, debris, stain, and plaque are removed.

10. _____ is a technique that uses a high-pressure stream of water and sodium bicarbonate to remove stain.

11. The _____ is the portion of the tooth that is visible in the mouth.

12. _____ is a type of sealant material supplied as a two-part system that is mixed together.

13. _____ is a technique used to remove plaque and stains from the coronal surfaces.

14. _____ stains cannot be removed by scaling or polishing.

15. _____ is a hard mineralized deposit on the teeth.

MULTIPLE CHOICE

16. Which of the following is an example of an extrinsic stain?
    a. tobacco stain
    b. dental fluorosis
    c. tetracycline antibiotic stain
    d. all of the above

17. Which of the following is an example of an intrinsic stain?
    a. pulpless teeth
    b. black stain
    c. food and drink
    d. all of the above

18. How do stains on the teeth occur?
    a. directly to the surface of the tooth
    b. embedded within the calculus and plaque deposits
    c. incorporated within the tooth structure
    d. all of the above

19. Which of the following is **not** an indication for dental sealants?
    a. deep pits and fissures
    b. recently erupted tooth
    c. occlusal surface decayed and needs a filling
    d. all of the above

20. Guidelines for sealant placement include:
    a. maintenance of a dry tooth surface
    b. preparing the tooth
    c. conditioning the tooth
    d. all of the above

Rubber Cup Coronal Polishing

Performance Objective

In states where coronal polishing by a dental assistant is legal, the student will demonstrate the proper procedure for a complete mouth coronal polish.

Grading Criteria

3 Student meets most of the criteria without assistance.

2 Student requires assistance to meet the stated criteria.

1 Student did not prepare accordingly for the stated criteria.

0 Not applicable.

Criteria	Peer	Self	Instructor	Comment
Preparation				
1. Gathered appropriate supplies.				
2. Prepared the patient and explained the procedure.				
3. Maintained the correct operator position and posture for each quadrant.				
4. Maintained adequate retraction and an appropriate fulcrum for each quadrant.				
5. Used the rubber polishing cup and abrasive with the proper polishing movements in all quadrants.				
6. Used the bristle brush and abrasive properly in all quadrants.				
7. Controlled the handpiece speed and pressure throughout the procedure while maintaining patient safety and comfort.				
8. Flossed between the patient's teeth.				
9. Rinsed the patient's mouth.				
10. Evaluated the coronal polish. Repeated steps as necessary.				
11. Maintained patient comfort and followed appropriate infection-control measures throughout the procedure.				

Total amount of points earned _____

Grade _____ *Instructor's initials* _____

Application of Dental Sealants

Performance Objective

In states where application of dental sealants by a dental assistant is legal, the student will demonstrate the proper procedure for applying pit and fissure sealants.

Grading Criteria

3 Student meets most of the criteria without assistance.

2 Student requires assistance to meet the stated criteria.

1 Student did not prepare accordingly for the stated criteria.

0 Not applicable.

Criteria	Peer	Self	Instructor	Comment
1. Gathered appropriate supplies.				
2. Seated the patient and explained the procedure.				
3. Polished the teeth to be treated.				
4. Used appropriate steps to prevent contamination by moisture or saliva.				
5. Placed the etching agent on the appropriate surfaces for the time specified by the manufacturer.				
6. Rinsed and dried the teeth and then verified the appearance of the etched surfaces. If the appearance was not satisfactory, etched the surfaces again.				
7. Placed the sealant on the etched surfaces.				
8. Light-cured the material according to the manufacturer's instructions.				
9. Checked the occlusion and made adjustments as necessary.				
10. Asked the dentist to evaluate the procedure before the patient was dismissed.				
11. Maintained patient comfort and followed appropriate infection-control measures throughout the procedure.				

Total amount of points earned _____

Grade _____ *Instructor's initials* _____

19 Instruments, Handpieces, and Accessories

TRUE/FALSE

_____ 1. Examination instruments allow the dentist to manually remove decay and prepare tooth structures.

_____ 2. Each hand instrument is made up of three parts: the handle, shank, and working end.

_____ 3. Instruments are organized on a tray to be used from right to left.

_____ 4. A rotary instrument includes the dental handpiece.

_____ 5. Plastic disposable prophy angles should be sterilized after use.

_____ 6. A long straight-shank bur will fit into the straight attachment of the low-speed handpiece.

_____ 7. Torque is the turning power of the instrument when pressure is applied.

_____ 8. The high-speed handpiece is equipped with a fiber-optic light.

_____ 9. Finishing burs are similar to carbide burs, but the blades are not as sharp and are farther apart.

_____ 10. A mandrel should be attached to the high-speed handpiece when using polishing disks.

MATCHING

_____ 11. Mouth mirror

_____ 12. Excavator

_____ 13. Amalgam carrier

_____ 14. Burnisher

_____ 15. Amalgam condenser

_____ 16. Hatchet

_____ 17. Cotton pliers

_____ 18. Hollenback carver

_____ 19. Diskoid/cleoid

_____ 20. Explorer

A. Carry, place, and remove items in the mouth

B. Used to examine healthy and diseased tooth structure

C. Carves amalgam on the occlusal surface

D. Smoothes the walls and floors of a tooth preparation

E. Removes soft dentin, debris, and decay

F. Carves amalgam at proximal surfaces

G. Carries amalgam to the prepared tooth

H. Smoothes amalgam on the occlusal surface

I. View, reflects light, retracts and protects tissue carver

J. Packs amalgam into the tooth preparation

21. List the four categories of dental hand instruments and describe their functions.

22. Fill in the name, number series, and use of each bur shape below.

A

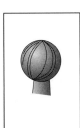

Name: _____

Number series: _____

Use: _____

C

Name: _____

Number series: _____

Use: _____

B

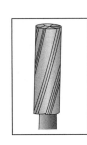

Name: _____

Number series: _____

Use: _____

D

Name: _____

Number series: _____

Use: _____

E

Name: _____

Number series: _____

Use: _____

F

Name: _____

Number series: _____

Use: _____

A-C, E, and **F** from Finkbeiner BL, Johnson CS: Mosby's comprehensive dental assisting, St Louis, 1955, Mosby.
D from Baum L, Phillips RW, Lund MR: Textbook of operative dentistry, ed 3, Philadelphia, 1995, Saunders.

Chapter **19 Instruments, Handpieces, and Accessories**

Identification of Dental Instruments for a Restorative Procedure

Performance Objective

The student will retrieve and organize the appropriate examination, hand-cutting, restorative, and accessory instruments and supplies for a restorative procedure.

Grading Criteria

3 Student meets most of the criteria without assistance.

2 Student requires assistance to meet the stated criteria.

1 Student did not prepare accordingly for the stated criteria.

0 Not applicable.

Criteria	Peer	Self	Instructor	Comment
Preparation				
1. Reviewed the patient record and determined the type of procedure and setup.				
2. Selected correct instruments for the procedure.				
3. Placed instruments in the appropriate order of use on the tray.				
4. Stated the use for each instrument and item placed on the tray setup.				

Total amount of points earned _____

Grade _____ *Instructor's initials* _____

Identifying and Attaching Handpieces and Rotary Instruments

Performance Objective

Given instructions for which size and/or type to select, the student will place and remove burs in a high-speed and a low-speed handpiece.

Grading Criteria

3 Student meets most of the criteria without assistance.

2 Student requires assistance to meet the stated criteria.

1 Student did not prepare accordingly for the stated criteria.

0 Not applicable.

Criteria	Peer	Self	Instructor	Comment
1. Attached the high-speed handpiece to the correct receptor on the dental unit.				
2. Attached the low-speed handpiece to the correct receptor on the dental unit.				
3. Attached the straight attachment, contra-angle attachment, and prophylaxis angle to the low-speed handpiece.				
4. Identified varying shapes of burs for the low-speed and high-speed handpiece.				
5. Selected the specified size and type of bur for the high-speed handpiece.				
6. Placed burs in the handpiece in accordance with the manufacturer's instructions.				
7. Removed burs from the handpiece in accordance with the manufacturer's instructions.				
8. Selected the specified size and type of bur for the low-speed handpiece.				
9. Placed the bur in the handpiece in accordance with the manufacturer's instructions.				
10. Removed the bur from the handpiece in accordance with the manufacturer's instructions.				

Total amount of points earned _____

Grade _____ *Instructor's initials* _____

20 Restorative Materials

TRUE/FALSE

_____ 1. Amalgam is referred to as an alloy.

_____ 2. IRM is the abbreviation for intermediate resin matrix.

_____ 3. ZOE is a dental material that can be considered for use as a temporary cement base, or as a permanent cement.

_____ 4. Luting agent is another term for composite resins.

_____ 5. Trituration is the process by which the mercury and alloy powder are mixed together.

_____ 6. Calcium hydroxide is a frequently selected type of cavity liner.

_____ 7. Etchant is a liquid or gel substance applied to the enamel or dentin surface for a specified period of time in preparation for the bonding material.

_____ 8. A base is placed on the gingival third of a prepared tooth before placement of the permanent restoration.

_____ 9. Zinc phosphate cement is exothermic in action when mixed.

_____ 10. Tooth whitening products are available in toothpaste, fluoride, floss, mouth rinses, and chewing gum.

MATCHING

Match the following restorative materials with their application.

_____ 11. Calcium hydroxide

_____ 12. Composite resin

_____ 13. Conditioner and/or etchant

_____ 14. Amalgam

_____ 15. Polycarboxylate cement

_____ 16. Bonding agent

_____ 17. Glass ionomer cement

_____ 18. Cavity varnish

A. Permanent restorative material for posterior teeth

B. Liner placed to regenerate and protect the pulp

C. Luting material for metal and ceramic restorations

D. Material that prepares tooth structure for bonding

E. Permanent restorative material for anterior teeth

F. Material that seals dentinal tubules

G. Material that creates retention between dental material and tooth structure

H. Luting agent for cast restoration and cementation of orthodontic bands

Match the properties of dental materials to their description.

_____ 19. Mechanical

_____ 20. Thermal

_____ 21. Electrical

_____ 22. Corrosive

_____ 23. Solubility

_____ 24. Application

A. The degree to which a substance will dissolve in a given amount of a wet environment

B. Reaction within a metal when it comes into contact with corrosive products

C. Specific steps in placing the material

D. A current takes place with the condition of metals interacting with saliva

E. Temperature change in the mouth

F. Biting and chewing in the posterior area of the mouth

SHORT ANSWER

25. Describe the composition of amalgam.

Mixing and Transferring Dental Amalgam

Performance Objective

The student will demonstrate the proper skills for mixing and transferring amalgam.

Grading Criteria

3 Student meets most of the criteria without assistance.

2 Student requires assistance to meet the stated criteria.

1 Student did not prepare accordingly for the stated criteria.

0 Not applicable.

Criteria	Peer	Self	Instructor	Comment
1. Selected the proper equipment and supplies.				
2. Activated the capsule using the activator.				
3. Placed the capsule in the amalgamator.				
4. Adjusted settings for the specific type of amalgam.				
5. Closed the cover on the amalgamator and began trituration.				
6. Removed the capsule and dispensed amalgam in the well.				
7. Filled the small end of the carrier and transferred to the dentist.				
8. Ensured that the carrier was directed toward the preparation.				
9. Continued delivery until the preparation was overfilled.				

Total amount of points earned _____

Grade _____ *Instructor's initials* _____

Preparing Composite Resin Materials

Performance Objective

The student will assemble the necessary supplies, then prepare composite resin for a restorative procedure.

Grading Criteria

3 Student meets most of the criteria without assistance.

2 Student requires assistance to meet the stated criteria.

1 Student did not prepare accordingly for the stated criteria.

0 Not applicable.

Criteria	Peer	Self	Instructor	Comment
1. Selected the proper equipment and supplies.				
2. Selected the shade of composite resin to match the tooth color using a shade guide and natural light.				
3. Expressed composite material onto treatment pad or in a light-protected well.				
4. Transferred the composite instrument and material to the dentist in the transfer zone.				
5. Had gauze available for the dentist to clean composite instrument.				
6. Had the curing light readied.				
7. When finished, cared for supplies and materials appropriately.				

Total amount of points earned _____

Grade _____ *Instructor's initials* _____

The Application of Calcium Hydroxide (Expanded Function)

Performance Objective

The student will assemble the necessary supplies and then correctly manipulate and place the cavity liner in a prepared tooth.

Grading Criteria

3 Student meets most of the criteria without assistance.

2 Student requires assistance to meet the stated criteria.

1 Student did not prepare accordingly for the stated criteria.

0 Not applicable.

Criteria	Peer	Self	Instructor	Comment
1. Selected the proper material and assembled the appropriate supplies.				
2. Dispensed small, equal amounts of the catalyst and base pastes onto the paper mixing pad.				
3. Used a circular motion to mix the material over a small area of the paper pad with the spatula.				
4. Used gauze to clean the spatula.				
5. With the tip of the applicator, picked up a small amount of the material, and applied a thin layer at the deepest area of the preparation.				
6. Used an explorer to remove any material from the enamel before drying.				
7. Cleaned and disinfected the equipment.				

Total amount of points earned _____

Grade _____ *Instructor's initials* _____

The Application of Dentin Sealer (Expanded Function)

Performance Objective

The student will assemble the necessary supplies and then correctly apply dentin sealer to a prepared tooth surface.

Grading Criteria

3 Student meets most of the criteria without assistance.

2 Student requires assistance to meet the stated criteria.

1 Student did not prepare accordingly for the stated criteria.

0 Not applicable.

Criteria	Peer	Self	Instructor	Comment
1. Selected the proper material and assembled the appropriate supplies.				
2. Rinsed the area with water and did not overdry.				
3. Applied the dentin sealer with the applicator over all areas of the dentin.				
4. Waited 30 seconds and dried the area thoroughly.				
5. Repeated application of sealer if sensitivity was a problem for the patient.				
6. Cleaned and disinfected the equipment.				

Total amount of points earned _____

Grade _____ *Instructor's initials* _____

Performance Objective

The student will assemble the necessary supplies and then correctly apply dental varnish to a prepared tooth surface.

Grading Criteria

3 Student meets most of the criteria without assistance.

2 Student requires assistance to meet the stated criteria.

1 Student did not prepare accordingly for the stated criteria.

0 Not applicable.

Criteria	Peer	Self	Instructor	Comment
1. Selected the proper material and assembled the appropriate supplies.				
2. Retrieved an applicator or sterile cotton pellets in cotton pliers.				
3. Opened the bottle of varnish and placed the tip of the applicator or cotton pellet into the liquid, making sure not to wet the cotton pliers.				
4. Replaced the cap on the bottle immediately.				
5. Placed a thin coating of the varnish on the walls, floor, and margin of the cavity preparation.				
6. Applied a second coat.				
7. Cleaned and disinfected the equipment.				

Total amount of points earned _____

Grade _____ Instructor's initials _____

Applying an Etchant Material (Expanded Function)

Performance Objective

The student will assemble the necessary supplies and then correctly apply etchant to a prepared tooth surface.

Grading Criteria

3 Student meets most of the criteria without assistance.

2 Student requires assistance to meet the stated criteria.

1 Student did not prepare accordingly for the stated criteria.

0 Not applicable.

Criteria	Peer	Self	Instructor	Comment
1. Selected the proper material and assembled the appropriate supplies.				
2. Used a dental dam or cotton rolls to isolate the prepared tooth.				
3. Ensured that the surface of the tooth structure was clean and free of any debris, plaque, or calculus before etching.				
4. Carefully dried (but did not desiccate) the surface.				
5. Applied etchant to the enamel or dentin.				
6. Etched the tooth structure for the time recommended by the manufacturer.				
7. After etching, thoroughly rinsed and dried the surface for 15 to 30 seconds.				
8. Ensured that the etched surface had a frosty-white appearance.				
9. When finished, cared for supplies and materials appropriately.				

Total amount of points earned _____

Grade _____ *Instructor's initials* _____

Applying a Bonding System (Expanded Function)

Performance Objective

The student will assemble the necessary supplies and then correctly apply a bonding system to a prepared tooth surface.

Grading Criteria

3 Student meets most of the criteria without assistance.

2 Student requires assistance to meet the stated criteria.

1 Student did not prepare accordingly for the stated criteria.

0 Not applicable.

Criteria	Peer	Self	Instructor	Comment
1. Selected the proper material and assembled the appropriate supplies.				
2. If a metal matrix band is required, prepared the band with either cavity varnish or wax before placement around the tooth.				
3. Etched the cavity preparation and the enamel margins according to the manufacturer's instructions.				
4. If a primer is part of the system, applied a primer to the entire preparation in one or multiple coats, depending on the manufacturer's instructions.				
5. Placed the dual-cured bonding resin in the entire cavity preparation and lightly air-thinned the material. The resin should appear unset or semiset.				
6. When finished, cared for supplies and materials appropriately.				

Total amount of points earned _____

Grade _____ *Instructor's initials* _____

Mixing Intermediate Restorative Materials

Performance Objective

The student will assemble the necessary supplies, then correctly manipulate the material for placement into a class I cavity preparation.

Grading Criteria

3 Student meets most of the criteria without assistance.

2 Student requires assistance to meet the stated criteria.

1 Student did not prepare accordingly for the stated criteria.

0 Not applicable.

Criteria	Peer	Self	Instructor	Comment
1. Selected the proper material and assembled the appropriate supplies.				
2. Dispensed materials in the proper sequence and quantity, then immediately recapped the containers.				
3. Incorporated the powder and liquid according to the manufacturer's instructions.				
4. Completed the mix within the appropriate working time.				
5. Ensured that, completed mix was the appropriate consistency for a temporary restoration.				
6. When finished, cared for supplies and materials appropriately.				

Total amount of points earned _____

Grade _____ *Instructor's initials* _____

Mixing Zinc Oxide–Eugenol (ZOE) for Permanent Cementation

Performance Objective

The student will assemble the necessary supplies and correctly manipulate ZOE for permanent cementation.

Grading Criteria

3 Student meets most of the criteria without assistance.

2 Student requires assistance to meet the stated criteria.

1 Student did not prepare accordingly for the stated criteria.

0 Not applicable.

Criteria	Peer	Self	Instructor	Comment
1. Selected the proper material and assembled the appropriate supplies.				
2. Measured the powder and placed it onto the mixing pad. Replaced the cap on the powder immediately.				
3. Dispensed the liquid near the powder on the mixing pad. Replaced the cap on the liquid container immediately.				
4. Incorporated the powder and liquid all at once and mixed it with the spatula for 30 seconds.				
5. After ensuring a puttylike consistency of the initial mix, mixed for an additional 30 seconds until it became more fluid for loading into a casting.				
6. Lined the crown with the permanent cement.				
7. Inverted the crown in the palm and readied for transfer.				
8. When finished, cared for supplies and materials appropriately.				

Total amount of points earned _____

Grade _____ *Instructor's initials* _____

Mixing Glass Ionomer for Permanent Cementation

Performance Objective

The student will assemble the necessary supplies and correctly manipulate the material for use in the cementation of a cast crown.

Grading Criteria

3 Student meets most of the criteria without assistance.

2 Student requires assistance to meet the stated criteria.

1 Student did not prepare accordingly for the stated criteria.

0 Not applicable.

Criteria	Peer	Self	Instructor	Comment
1. Selected the proper material and assembled the appropriate supplies.				
2. Dispensed the manufacturer's recommended proportion of the *liquid* on one half of the paper pad.				
3. Dispensed the manufacturer's recommended proportion of the *powder* on the other half of the pad; this is usually divided into two or three increments.				
4. Incorporated the powder and liquid for the recommended mixing time until the material had a glossy appearance.				
5. Lined the inside of the crown with cement.				
6. Turned the casting over in the palm and transferred it to the dentist.				
7. Transferred a cotton roll so the patient could bite down on it to help seat the crown and displace the excess cement.				
8. When finished, cared for supplies and materials appropriately.				

Total amount of points earned _____

Grade _____ *Instructor's initials* _____

Mixing Zinc Phosphate for Permanent Cementation

Performance Objective

The student will assemble the necessary supplies and correctly manipulate the material for use in the cementation of a cast crown.

Grading Criteria

3 Student meets most of the criteria without assistance.

2 Student requires assistance to meet the stated criteria.

1 Student did not prepare accordingly for the stated criteria.

0 Not applicable.

Criteria	Peer	Self	Instructor	Comment
Preparing the Mix				
1. Selected the proper material and assembled the appropriate supplies.				
2. Cooled the glass slab for mixing.				
3. Dispensed the powder toward one end of the slab and the liquid at the opposite end. Recapped the containers.				
4. Divided the powder into small increments as directed by the manufacturer.				
5. Incorporated each powder increment into the liquid, beginning with smaller increments.				
6. Spatulated the mix thoroughly, using broad strokes or a figure-eight movement over a large area of the slab.				
7. Tested the material for appropriate cementation consistency. (The cement should string up and break about 1 inch from the slab.)				
Placing Cement in the Casting				
1. Held the casting with the inner portion facing upward.				
2. Retrieved the cement onto the spatula. Scraped the edge of the spatula along the margin to cause the cement to flow from the spatula into the casting.				
3. Placed the tip of the spatula or a black spoon into the bulk of the cement and moved the material so that it covered all internal walls with a thin lining of cement.				
4. Turned the casting over in the palm and transferred it to the dentist.				
5. Transferred a cotton roll so the patient could bite down on it to help seat the crown and displace the excess cement.				
6. When finished, cared for supplies and materials appropriately.				

Total amount of points earned _____

Grade _____ *Instructor's initials* _____

Mixing Polycarboxylate for Permanent Cementation

Performance Objective

The student will assemble the necessary supplies and correctly manipulate the material for use in cementation.

Grading Criteria

3 Student meets most of the criteria without assistance.

2 Student requires assistance to meet the stated criteria.

1 Student did not prepare accordingly for the stated criteria.

0 Not applicable.

Criteria	Peer	Self	Instructor	Comment
For Cementation				
1. Selected the proper material and assembled the appropriate supplies.				
2. Gently shook the powder to fluff the ingredients.				
3. Measured the powder onto the mixing pad and immediately recapped the container.				
4. Dispensed the liquid and then recapped the container.				
5. Used the flat side of the spatula to incorporate all the powder quickly into the liquid at one time. The mix must be completed within 30 seconds.				
6. Ensured that the mix was somewhat thick with a shiny, glossy surface.				
7. Lined the inside of the crown with cement.				
8. Turned the casting over in the palm and transferred it to the dentist.				
9. Transferred a cotton roll so the patient could bite down on it to help seat the crown and displace the excess cement.				
10. When finished, cared for supplies and materials appropriately.				

Total amount of points earned _____

Grade _____ *Instructor's initials* _____

21 | Restorative Procedures

TRUE/FALSE

_____ 1. Esthetic dentistry is primarily devoted to improving the appearance of teeth.

_____ 2. The purpose of cavity preparation is to remove decay and a small amount of healthy tooth structure.

_____ 3. Universal matrix bands are made of a soft latex material.

_____ 4. Before assembling the matrix into the retainer, you must varnish the band for use.

_____ 5. A veneer is a thin layer of tooth-colored material bonded on the facial surface of a tooth.

_____ 6. A wedge is placed into the embrasure to hold the matrix band firmly against the margin of a preparation.

_____ 7. When a tooth is badly decayed, the placement of retentive pins along with a bonding material may be required.

_____ 8. Vital bleaching is a technique involved in the whitening of the pulpal portion of the teeth.

_____ 9. The dentist will commonly use hand instruments over rotary instruments to prepare tooth structure and retentive grooves in the preparation.

_____ 10. A clear plastic matrix strip is the matrix of choice for Class III and IV anterior restorations.

MATCHING

Match the type of restoration to Black's classification of cavities.

_____ 11. Incisal edge composite   A. Class VI

_____ 12. Occlusal amalgam   B. Class II

_____ 13. Mesial-incisal composite   C. Class I

_____ 14. Distal composite   D. Class III

_____ 15. Mesial-occlusal-distal amalgam   E. Class IV

         F. Class V

_____ 16. Gingival-third composite

SHORT ANSWER

17. Describe the conditions that would require restorative dental treatment.

18. Describe the conditions that would require esthetic dental treatment.

Assembling the Matrix Band and Universal Retainer

Performance Objective

The student will demonstrate the proper technique for assembling a matrix band and Tofflemire retainer for each quadrant of the dental arch.

Grading Criteria

3 Student meets most of the criteria without assistance.

2 Student requires assistance to meet the stated criteria.

1 Student did not prepare accordingly for the stated criteria.

0 Not applicable.

Criteria	Peer	Self	Instructor	Comment
1. Gathered the appropriate supplies.				
2. Stated which guide slot would be used for each quadrant.				
3. Determined the tooth to be treated and selected the appropriate band.				
4. Placed the middle of the band on the paper pad and burnished the band with a ball burnisher.				
5. Held the retainer so that the diagonal slot was visible and turned the outer knob clockwise until the end of the spindle was visible in the diagonal slot in the vise.				
6. Turned the inner knob counterclockwise until the vise moved next to the guide slots and the retainer was ready to receive the matrix band.				
7. Identified the occlusal and gingival aspects of the matrix band and brought the ends of the band together to form a loop.				
8. Placed the occlusal edge of the band into the retainer first and then guided the band between the correct guide slots.				
9. Locked the band in the vise.				
10. Used the handle end of the mouth mirror to open and round the loop of the band.				
11. Adjusted the size of the loop to fit the selected tooth.				

Total amount of points earned _____

Grade _____ *Instructor's initials* _____

Assisting in an Amalgam Restoration

Performance Objective

The student will demonstrate the proper techniques when assisting with the preparation, placement, and finishing of an amalgam restoration.

Grading Criteria

3 Student meets most of the criteria without assistance.

2 Student requires assistance to meet the stated criteria.

1 Student did not prepare accordingly for the stated criteria.

0 Not applicable.

Criteria	Peer	Self	Instructor	Comment
1. Gathered the appropriate setup.				
2. Dental materials were placed and readied.				
3. Assisted during administration of topical and local anesthetic solution.				
4. Assisted in placement of the dental dam or other moisture-control devices.				
Preparing the Tooth				
1. Transferred the mirror and explorer.				
2. During cavity preparation, used the HVE and air-water syringe, adjusted the light, and retracted as necessary to maintain a clear field.				
3. Transferred the explorer, excavators, and hand-cutting instruments as needed throughout cavity preparation.				
Placing the Matrix Band and Wedge (if required)				
1. Prepared the universal retainer and matrix band according to preparation.				
2. Either assisted in placement or performed complete placement of the matrix band.				
3. Assisted in placement or performed complete insertion of wedges using #110 pliers.				
Placing Dental Materials				
1. Rinsed and dried the preparation for evaluation.				
2. Mixed and transferred the base, liner, sealer, etchant, and bonding materials in the proper sequence.				

Criteria	Peer	Self	Instructor	Comment
Mixing the Amalgam				
1. Activated the capsule, placed it in the amalgamator, and set the correct time for trituration.				
2. Placed mixed amalgam in the well.				
3. Reassembled the capsule and discarded it properly.				
Placing, Condensing, and Carving the Amalgam				
1. Filled the amalgam carrier and transferred it to the dentist.				
2. Transferred restorative instruments as needed to the dentist.				
3. Transferred the carving instruments.				
4. Assisted with removal of the wedge, retainer, matrix band, and dental dam.				
5. Assisted during final carving and occlusal adjustment.				
6. Gave postoperative instructions to the patient.				
7. Maintained patient comfort and followed appropriate infection-control measures throughout the procedure.				
8. When finished, cared for supplies and materials appropriately.				

Total amount of points earned _____

Grade _____ *Instructor's initials* _____

Performance Objective

The student will demonstrate the proper techniques when assisting with the preparation, placement, and finishing of a composite restoration.

Grading Criteria

3 Student meets most of the criteria without assistance.

2 Student requires assistance to meet the stated criteria.

1 Student did not prepare accordingly for the stated criteria.

0 Not applicable.

Criteria	Peer	Self	Instructor	Comment
1. Gathered the appropriate setup.				
2. Dental materials were placed and readied.				
3. Assisted during administration of the topical and local anesthetic solutions.				
4. Assisted in selection of the shade of composite material.				
5. Assisted in placement of the dental dam or other moisture-control devices.				
Preparing the Tooth				
1. Transferred the mirror and explorer.				
2. During cavity preparation, used the HVE and air-water syringe, adjusted the light, and retracted as necessary to maintain a clear field.				
3. Transferred the explorer, excavators, and hand-cutting instruments as needed throughout cavity preparation.				
Placing the Matrix Band and Wedge (if required)				
1. Prepared a clear strip and wedge according to the preparation.				
2. Either assisted in placement or performed complete placement of the matrix band.				
3. Assisted in placement or performed complete insertion of wedges using #110 pliers.				
Placing Dental Materials				
1. Rinsed and dried the preparation for evaluation.				
2. Mixed and transferred the base, liner, sealer, etchant, and bonding materials in proper sequence.				

Criteria	Peer	Self	Instructor	Comment
Preparing the Composite				
1. Dispensed the composite material on the paper pad and transferred it to the dentist.				
2. Transferred restorative instruments as needed to the dentist.				
3. Assisted in light-curing of the material.				
Finishing the Restoration				
1. Assisted with the transfer of burs or diamonds for the high-speed handpiece.				
2. Transferred finishing strips.				
3. Assisted with removal of the wedge, matrix band, and dental dam.				
4. Assisted during final polishing and occlusal adjustment.				
5. Gave postoperative instructions to the patient.				
6. Maintained patient comfort and followed appropriate infection-control measures throughout the procedure.				
7. When finished, cared for supplies and materials appropriately.				

Total amount of points earned _____

Grade _____ *Instructor's initials* _____

22 Impression Materials and Laboratory Procedures

TRUE/FALSE

_____ 1. Impression trays that are supplied as quadrant trays cover half of the arch.

_____ 2. When an impression is poured up, it creates a negative reproduction of the teeth and the surrounding structures.

_____ 3. Alginate is an irreversible hydrocolloid.

_____ 4. The water-to-powder ratio for mixing alginate is one scoop of powder to the second "measure line" of water.

_____ 5. A diagnostic cast is the model that is fabricated from the impression.

_____ 6. Dental stone is weaker than model plaster.

_____ 7. The way casts are trimmed is by the use of a laboratory handpiece.

_____ 8. Heavy body impression material is the most commonly used tray material.

_____ 9. Another term for occlusal registration is bite registration.

_____ 10. The two most common ways to mix final impression materials are the mixing of two pastes and the use of a triturator.

MATCHING

Match the type of impression material with its use (answer choices can be used more than once).

_____ 11. Alginate

_____ 12. Polysulfide

_____ 13. Wax

_____ 14. Condensation silicone

_____ 15. Polyether

A. Preliminary impression

B. Final impression

C. Occlusal registration

SHORT ANSWER

16. List the five factors that influence the setting of gypsum.

17. List the two types of impression trays and give their characteristics.

227

Mixing Alginate Impression Material

Performance Objective

The student will mix alginate impression material.

Grading Criteria

3 Student meets most of the criteria without assistance.

2 Student requires assistance to meet the stated criteria.

1 Student did not prepare accordingly for the stated criteria.

0 Not applicable.

Criteria	Peer	Self	Instructor	Comment
1. Gathered appropriate supplies.				
2. Placed the appropriate amount of water into the bowl.				
3. Shook the can of alginate to "fluff" the contents. After fluffing, carefully lifted the lid to prevent the particles from flying into the air.				
4. Sifted the powder into the water and used the spatula to mix with a stirring action to wet the powder until it has all been moistened.				
5. Firmly spread the alginate between the spatula and the side of the rubber bowl.				
6. Mixed with the spatula for the appropriate time until the mixture appeared smooth and creamy.				
7. Wiped the alginate mix into one mass on the inside edge of the bowl.				
8. When finished, cared for supplies and materials appropriately.				

Total amount of points earned _____

Grade _____ *Instructor's initials* _____

Taking a Mandibular or a Maxillary Preliminary Impression (Expanded Function)

Performance Objective

The student will take a mandibular and maxillary alginate impression of diagnostic quality.

Grading Criteria

3 Student meets most of the criteria without assistance.

2 Student requires assistance to meet the stated criteria.

1 Student did not prepare accordingly for the stated criteria.

0 Not applicable.

Criteria	Peer	Self	Instructor	Comment
1. Gathered all necessary supplies.				
2. Seated and prepared the patient.				
3. Explained the procedure to the patient.				
4. Selected and prepared the mandibular impression tray.				
5. Measured two measures of room-temperature water with two scoops of alginate and mixed the material.				
Loading the Mandibular Impression Tray				
1. Gathered half of the alginate in the bowl onto the spatula, then wiped alginate into one side of the tray from the lingual side. Quickly pressed the material down to the base of the tray.				
2. Gathered the remaining half of the alginate in the bowl onto the spatula and then loaded the other side of the tray in the same way.				
3. Smoothed the surface of the alginate by wiping a moistened finger along the surface.				
Seating the Mandibular Impression Tray				
1. Placed additional material over the occlusal surfaces of the mandibular teeth.				
2. Retracted the patient's cheek with the index finger.				
3. Turned the tray slightly sideways when placing it into the mouth.				
4. Centered the tray over the teeth.				
5. Seated the tray from the posterior border first.				
6. Instructed the patient to breathe normally while the material set.				
7. Observed the alginate around the tray to determine when the material had set.				

Criteria	Peer	Self	Instructor	Comment
Removing the Mandibular Impression				
1. Placed fingers on top of the impression tray and gently broke the seal between the impression and the peripheral tissues by moving the inside of the patient's cheeks or lips with the finger.				
2. Grasped the handle of the tray with the thumb and index finger and used a firm lifting motion to break the seal.				
3. Snapped up the tray and impression from the dentition.				
4. Instructed the patient to rinse with water to remove excess alginate material.				
5. Evaluated the impression for accuracy.				
Loading the Maxillary Impression Tray				
1. For a maxillary impression, mixed three measures of water and three scoops of powder.				
2. Loaded the maxillary tray in one large increment and used a wiping motion to fill the tray from the posterior end.				
3. Placed the bulk of the material toward the anterior palatal area of the tray.				
4. Moistened fingertips with tap water and smoothed the surface of the alginate.				
Seating the Maxillary Impression Tray				
1. Used the index finger to retract the patient's cheek.				
2. Turned the tray slightly sideways to position the tray into the mouth.				
3. Centered the tray over the patient's teeth.				
4. Seated the posterior border (back) of the tray up against the posterior border of the hard palate to form a seal.				
5. Directed the anterior portion of the tray upward over the teeth.				
6. Gently lifted the patient's lips out of the way as the tray was seated.				
7. Checked the posterior border of the tray to ensure that no material was flowing into the patient's throat. If necessary, wiped excess material away with a cotton-tipped applicator.				
8. Held the tray firmly in place while the alginate set.				

Criteria	Peer	Self	Instructor	Comment
Removing the Maxillary Impression				
1. To prevent injury to the impression and the patient's teeth, placed a finger along the lateral borders of the tray to push down and break the palatal seal.				
2. Used a straight, downward snapping motion to remove the tray from the teeth.				
3. Instructed the patient to rinse with water to remove any excess alginate impression material.				
Caring for Alginate Impressions				
1. Gently rinsed the impression under cold tap water to remove any blood or saliva.				
2. Sprayed the impression with an approved disinfectant.				
3. Wrapped the impression in a damp paper towel and stored it in a covered container or plastic biohazard bag labeled with the patient's name.				
Before Dismissing the Patient				
1. Examined the patient's mouth for any remaining fragments of alginate and removed them using an explorer and dental floss.				
2. Used a moist facial tissue to remove any alginate from the patient's face and lips.				

Total amount of points earned _____

Grade _____ *Instructor's initials* _____

Chapter **22** **Impression Materials and Laboratory Procedures**

Mixing Dental Plaster

Performance Objective

The student will mix dental plaster in preparation for pouring a dental model.

Grading Criteria

3 Student meets most of the criteria without assistance.

2 Student requires assistance to meet the stated criteria.

1 Student did not prepare accordingly for the stated criteria.

0 Not applicable.

Criteria	Peer	Self	Instructor	Comment
1. Gathered appropriate supplies.				
2. Measured 45 mL of room-temperature water into a clean rubber mixing bowl.				
3. Weighed out 100 g of dental plaster.				
4. Added the powder to the water in steady increments. Allowed the powder to settle into the water for about 30 seconds.				
5. Used the spatula to incorporate the powder slowly into the water.				
6. Achieved a smooth and creamy mix in about 20 seconds.				
7. Turned the vibrator to low or medium speed and placed the bowl of plaster mix on the vibrator platform.				
8. Lightly pressed and rotated the bowl on the vibrator until air bubbles rose to the surface.				
9. Completed mixing and vibration of the plaster in *2 minutes or less*.				
10. When finished, cared for supplies and materials appropriately.				

Note: Mandibular and maxillary impressions have already been taken.

Total amount of points earned _____

Grade _____ Instructor's initials _____

Chapter **22** **Impression Materials and Laboratory Procedures**

Performance Objective

The student will pour a maxillary and mandibular dental model using the inverted-pour method.

Grading Criteria

3 Student meets most of the criteria without assistance.

2 Student requires assistance to meet the stated criteria.

1 Student did not prepare accordingly for the stated criteria.

0 Not applicable.

Criteria	Peer	Self	Instructor	Comment
1. Gathered the appropriate supplies.				
Preparing the Impression				
1. Used air to remove excess moisture from the impression.				
2. Used a lab knife or lab cutters to remove any excess impression material that will interfere with the pouring of the model.				
Pouring the Mandibular Model and Base				
1. Mixed the plaster, then set the vibrator at low to medium speed.				
2. Held the impression tray by the handle and placed the edge of the tray on the vibrator.				
3. Placed small increments of plaster in the impression near the most posterior tooth.				
4. Continued to place small increments in the same area as the first increment and allowed the plaster to flow toward the anterior teeth.				
5. Turned the tray on its side to provide the continuous flow of material forward into each tooth impression.				
6. When all the teeth in the impression were covered, added larger increments until the entire impression was filled.				
7. Placed the additional material onto a glass slab (or tile) and shaped the base to approximately 2 by 2 inches and 1 inch thick.				
8. Inverted the impression onto the new mix without pushing the impression into the base.				
9. Used a spatula to smooth the plaster base mix up onto the margins of the initial pour.				

Criteria	Peer	Self	Instructor	Comment
Pouring the Maxillary Cast				
1. Repeated steps 3 to 5 using clean equipment for the fresh mix of plaster.				
2. Placed a small increment of plaster at the posterior area of the impression. Guided the material as it flows down into the impression of the most posterior tooth.				
3. Continued to place small increments in the same area as the first increment and allowed the plaster to flow toward the anterior teeth.				
4. Rotated the tray on its side to provide the continuous flow of material into each tooth impression.				
5. When all teeth in the impression were covered, added larger increments until the entire impression was filled.				
6. Placed the mix onto a glass slab (or tile) and shaped the base to approximately 2 by 2 inches or 1 inch thick.				
7. Inverted the impression onto the new mix.				
8. Used a spatula to smooth the stone base mix up onto the margins of the initial pour.				
9. Placed the impression tray on the base so that the handle and occlusal plane of the teeth on the cast were parallel with the surface of the glass slab (or tile).				
Separating the Cast from the Impression				
1. Waited 45 to 60 minutes after the base was poured before separating the impression from the model.				
2. Used the laboratory knife to gently separate the margins of the tray.				
3. Applied firm, straight, upward pressure on the handle of the tray to remove the impression.				
4. Pulled the tray handle straight up from the model.				
5. Readied the models for trimming and polishing.				
6. When finished, cared for supplies and materials appropriately.				

Total amount of points earned _____

Grade _____ *Instructor's initials* _____

Performance Objective

The student will trim and finish a set of dental models to be used for diagnostic purposes.

Grading Criteria

3 Student meets most of the criteria without assistance.

2 Student requires assistance to meet the stated criteria.

1 Student did not prepare accordingly for the stated criteria.

0 Not applicable.

Criteria	Peer	Self	Instructor	Comment
1. Gathered appropriate supplies.				
Preparing the Model				
1. Soaked the art portion of the model in a bowl of water for at least 5 minutes.				
Trimming the Maxillary Model				
1. Placed the maxillary model on a flat countertop with the teeth setting on the table.				
2. Measured up 1¼ inches from the counter and drew a line around the model.				
3. Turned on the trimmer, held the model firmly against the trimmer, and trimmed the bottom of the base to the line drawn.				
4. Drew a line ¼ inch behind the maxillary tuberosities. With the base flat on the trimmer, removed excess plaster in the posterior area of the model to the marked line.				
5. Drew a line through the center of the occlusal ridges on one side of the model. Measured out ¼ inch from the line and drew a line parallel to the line drawn.				
6. Repeated these measurements on the other side of the model.				
7. Trimmed the sides of the cast to the lines drawn.				
8. Trimmed maxillary heel cuts by drawing a line behind the tuberosity that was perpendicular to the opposite canine.				
9. Made the final cut by drawing a line from the canine to the midline at an angle (completed this on both sides and trimmed to the line).				

Criteria	Peer	Self	Instructor	Comment
Trimming the Mandibular Model				
1. Occluded the mandibular model with the maxillary model using the wax bite.				
2. With the mandibular base on the trimmer, trimmed the posterior portion of the mandibular model until even with the maxillary model.				
3. Placed the models upside down (maxillary base on the table), measured 3 inches from the surface up, and marked a line around the base of the mandibular model.				
4. Trimmed the mandibular model base to the line drawn.				
5. With the models in occlusion with the wax bite, placed the mandibular model on the trimmer, and trimmed the lateral cuts to match the maxillary lateral cuts.				
6. Trimmed the back and heel cuts to match the maxillary heel cuts.				
7. Checked that the mandibular anterior cut was a rounded circle from the mandibular canine to the mandibular canine.				
Finishing the Model				
1. Mixed a slurry of gypsum and filled any voids.				
2. Used a laboratory knife to remove any extra gypsum that appeared as beads on the occlusion or model.				
3. When finished, cared for supplies and materials appropriately.				

Total amount of points earned _____

Grade _____ Instructor's initials _____

Mixing a Two-Paste Final Impression Material

Performance Objective

The student will prepare and mix a two-paste final impression material.

Grading Criteria

3 Student meets most of the criteria without assistance.

2 Student requires assistance to meet the stated criteria.

1 Student did not prepare accordingly for the stated criteria.

0 Not applicable.

Criteria	Peer	Self	Instructor	Comment
1. Gathered appropriate supplies.				
Preparing Light-Bodied Syringe Material				
1. Dispensed approximately 1½ to 2 inches of equal lengths of the base and catalyst of the light-bodied material onto the top third of the pad, ensuring that the materials were not too close to each other.				
2. Wiped the tube openings clean with gauze and recapped immediately.				
3. Placed the tip of the spatula blade into the catalyst and base and mixed in a swirling direction for approximately 5 seconds.				
4. Gathered the material onto the flat portion of the spatula and placed it on a clean area of the pad, preferably the center.				
5. Spatulated smoothly, wiping back and forth and trying to use only one side of the spatula during the mixing process.				
6. To obtain a more homogenous mix, picked the material up by the spatula blade and wiped it onto the pad.				
7. Gathered the material together, took the syringe tube, and began "cookie cutting" the material into the syringe. Inserted the plunger and expressed a small amount of the material to ensure that it was in working order.				
8. Transferred the syringe to the dentist, ensuring that the tip of the syringe was directed toward the tooth.				

Criteria	Peer	Self	Instructor	Comment
Preparing Heavy-Bodied Tray Material				
1. Dispensed equal lengths of the base and catalyst of the heavy-bodied material on the top third of the pad for a quadrant tray.				
2. Placed the tip of the spatula blade into the catalyst and base and mixed in a swirling direction for approximately 5 seconds.				
3. Gathered the material onto the flat portion of the spatula and placed it on a clean area of the pad.				
4. Spatulated smoothly, wiping back and forth using only one side of the spatula during the mixing process.				
5. To get a more homogenous mix, picked the material up by the spatula blade and wiped it on the pad.				
6. Gathered the bulk of the material with the spatula and loaded the material into the tray.				
7. Using tip of the spatula, spread the material evenly from one end of the tray to the other without picking up the material.				
8. Retrieved the syringe from the dentist and transferred the tray, ensuring that the dentist could grasp the handle of the tray properly.				
9. When finished, cared for supplies and materials appropriately.				

Total amount of points earned _____

Grade _____ *Instructor's initials* _____

Preparing an Automix Final Impression Material

Performance Objective

The student will prepare an automix final impression material.

Grading Criteria

3 Student meets most of the criteria without assistance.

2 Student requires assistance to meet the stated criteria.

1 Student did not prepare accordingly for the stated criteria.

0 Not applicable.

Criteria	Peer	Self	Instructor	Comment
1. Gathered appropriate supplies.				
2. Loaded the extruder with dual cartridges of the base and the catalyst of light-bodied material.				
3. Removed the caps from the tube and extruded a small amount of unmixed material onto the gauze pad.				
4. Attached a mixing tip on the extruder along with a syringe tip for the light-bodied application by the dentist.				
5. When the dentist signaled, began squeezing the trigger until the material reached the tip.				
6. Transferred the extruder to the dentist, directing the tip toward the area of the impression.				
7. Placed the heavy-bodied cartridges in the extruder, expressing a small amount as before with the light body. Attached the mixing tip to the cartridge.				
8. When the dentist signaled, began squeezing the trigger, mixing the heavy-bodied material.				
9. Loaded the impression tray with heavy-bodied material, making sure not to trap air into the material.				
10. Transferred the tray, ensuring that the dentist can grasp the handle of the tray.				
11. Disinfected the impression, placed it in a biohazard bag, labeled it with the patient's name, and readied it for the laboratory.				

Total amount of points earned _____

Grade _____ *Instructor's initials* _____

23 Prosthodontics

TRUE/FALSE

_____ 1. Gingival retraction cord permanently moves the gingival tissue and widens the sulcus.

_____ 2. Provisional coverage is also known as temporary coverage.

_____ 3. Prosthodontics encompasses two areas of dentistry: fixed and removable prosthodontics.

_____ 4. To ensure an exact color match, many dentists prefer to check the shade using fluorescent lighting.

_____ 5. A core buildup is made of amalgam or a specific core material.

_____ 6. A removable partial denture replaces all of the teeth in an arch.

_____ 7. Anterior teeth are the recommended teeth for abutments of a partial.

_____ 8. Pressure points are areas within the tissue portion of the denture that could possibly rub the patient's tissue.

_____ 9. The use of gingival retraction cord is not required when taking a final impression for a denture.

_____ 10. An immediate denture is placed immediately following the placement of an implant.

MATCHING

Match the following types of prostheses to their description.

_____ 11. Fixed prosthesis that covers a portion of the occlusal and proximal surfaces of a tooth

_____ 12. Removable prosthesis that replaces all of the teeth in one arch

_____ 13. Full metal crown with an outer surface covered with a thin layer of tooth-colored material

_____ 14. Prosthesis cemented in place that covers the anatomic portion of an individual tooth

_____ 15. Removable prosthesis that replaces one or more teeth in same arch

_____ 16. A prosthesis cemented in place that replaces one or more adjacent teeth in the same arch

_____ 17. Thin shell of tooth-colored material bonded on the facial surface of anterior teeth

A. Porcelain fused to metal

B. Fixed bridge

C. Veneer

D. Complete denture

E. Full crown

F. Partial denture

G. Onlay

18. List the indications for a partial denture.

19. List the indications for a complete denture.

20. Describe the specific objective for provisional coverage.

Placing and Removing Gingival Retraction Cord (Expanded Function)

Performance Objective

The student will demonstrate the proper technique for placing, packing, and removing gingival retraction cord.

Grading Criteria

3 Student meets most of the criteria without assistance.

2 Student requires assistance to meet the stated criteria.

1 Student did not prepare accordingly for the stated criteria.

0 Not applicable.

Criteria	Peer	Self	Instructor	Comment
Preparing the Tooth and Cord				
1. Gathered the appropriate setup.				
2. Rinsed and gently dried the prepared tooth and isolated the quadrant with cotton rolls.				
3. Cut a piece of retraction cord 1 to 1½ inches in length, depending on the size and type of tooth under preparation.				
4. Formed a loose loop of the cord and placed the cord in the cotton pliers.				
Placing the Cord				
1. Slipped the loop of the retraction cord over the tooth so that the overlapping ends were on the facial-buccal surface.				
2. Laid the cord into the sulcus. Then used the packing instrument, and working in a clockwise direction, packed the cord gently but firmly into the sulcus.				
3. Used a gentle rocking movement of the instrument as it moved forward to the next loose section of retraction cord. Repeated this action until the length of cord was packed in place.				
4. Overlapped the working end of the cord where it met the first end of the cord. Tucked the ends into the sulcus on the facial aspect.				
5. Left the cord in place for no longer than 5 to 7 minutes. During this time, advised the patient to remain still and kept the area dry.				
Removing the Cord				
1. Grasped the end of the retraction cord with cotton pliers and removed the cord in a counterclockwise direction.				
2. If instructed by the operator, gently dried the area and placed fresh cotton rolls.				

Total amount of points earned _____

Grade _____ *Instructor's initials* _____

Assisting in a Crown and Bridge Preparation

Performance Objective

The student will demonstrate the proper technique when assisting the preparation for a crown and bridge restoration.

Grading Criteria

3 Student meets most of the criteria without assistance.

2 Student requires assistance to meet the stated criteria.

1 Student did not prepare accordingly for the stated criteria.

0 Not applicable.

Criteria	Peer	Self	Instructor	Comment
1. Gathered the appropriate setup.				
2. Took a preliminary impression for making the provisional coverage.				
3. Assisted during the administration of topical and local anesthesia.				
4. Throughout the preparation, maintained a clear, well-lighted operating field.				
5. Anticipated the dentist's needs. Transferred instruments and changed burs as necessary.				
6. Assisted or placed gingival retraction cord.				
7. Assisted in mixing the impression material and taking the final impression.				
8. Assisted or fabricated the provisional coverage.				
9. Temporarily cemented the provisional coverage.				
10. Prepared the case to be sent to the laboratory.				
11. Maintained patient comfort and followed appropriate infection-control measures throughout the procedure.				

Total amount of points earned _____

Grade _____ *Instructor's initials* _____

Fabricating and Cementing a Custom Acrylic Provisional Crown (Expanded Function)

Performance Objective

The student will demonstrate the proper technique for preparing and placing temporary coverage for a tooth prepared to receive a crown.

Grading Criteria

3 Student meets most of the criteria without assistance.

2 Student requires assistance to meet the stated criteria.

1 Student did not prepare accordingly for the stated criteria.

0 Not applicable.

Criteria	Peer	Self	Instructor	Comment
Preliminary Impression				
1. Gathered the appropriate setup.				
2. Obtained the preliminary impression.				
Create the Provisional Coverage				
1. Isolated and dried the prepared tooth.				
2. Prepared provisional material according to the manufacturer's directions.				
3. Placed the material in the impression in the area of the prepared tooth. Returned the impression to the mouth and allowed it to set for 2 minutes or longer.				
4. Removed the impression from the patient's mouth and then removed the provisional coverage from the impression.				
5. Used acrylic burs to trim the temporary coverage.				
6. Cured the provisional coverage according to the manufacturer's instructions.				
7. After curing, removed any excess material with finishing diamonds, disks, or finishing burs.				
8. Checked the occlusion and made any adjustments using the laboratory burs and disks on the provisional outside of the mouth.				
9. Completed final polishing using rubber disks and polishing lathe and pumice.				

Criteria	Peer	Self	Instructor	Comment
Cementation				
1. Mixed the temporary cement and filled the crown.				
2. Seated the provisional coverage and allowed the cement to set.				
3. Removed any excess cement and checked the occlusion.				
4. Had dentist check and evaluate the procedure.				
5. Provided the patient with home-care instructions.				
6. Maintained patient comfort and followed appropriate infection-control measures throughout the procedure.				

Total amount of points earned _____

Grade _____ *Instructor's initials* _____

Assisting in the Delivery and Cementation of a Cast Restoration

Performance Objective

The student will demonstrate the proper technique when assisting during the cementation of a crown and bridge restoration.

Grading Criteria

3 Student meets most of the criteria without assistance.

2 Student requires assistance to meet the stated criteria.

1 Student did not prepare accordingly for the stated criteria.

0 Not applicable.

Criteria	Peer	Self	Instructor	Comment
1. Determined in advance that the case had been returned from the laboratory.				
2. Gathered the appropriate setup.				
3. Assisted during the administration of topical and local anesthesia.				
4. Assisted during the removal of provisional coverage. (In a state where it is legal, removed the provisional coverage.)				
5. Anticipated the dentist's needs while the casting was tried in and adjusted.				
6. Assisted with or placed cotton rolls to isolate the quadrant and keep the area dry.				
7. Assisted during placement of cavity varnish or desensitizer.				
8. At a signal from the dentist, mixed the cement, lined the internal surface of the casting with a thin coating of cement, and transferred the prepared crown to the dentist.				
9. Provided home-care instructions to the patient.				
10. Maintained patient comfort and followed appropriate infection-control measures throughout the procedure.				

Total amount of points earned _____

Grade _____ *Instructor's initials* _____

Assisting in the Delivery of the Partial and Complete Denture

Performance Objective

The student will demonstrate the proper technique when assisting with the preparation and placement of a complete and/or partial denture.

Grading Criteria

3 Student meets most of the criteria without assistance.

2 Student requires assistance to meet the stated criteria.

1 Student did not prepare accordingly for the stated criteria.

0 Not applicable.

Criteria	Peer	Self	Instructor	Comment
Preliminary Visits				
1. Exposed radiographs as requested.				
2. Prepared diagnostic casts as requested.				
3. If necessary, prepared a custom tray.				
Preparation Visit				
1. Assisted during preparation of the teeth.				
2. Assisted in obtaining the final impression, opposing arch impression, and intraoral occlusal registration.				
3. Disinfected the completed impressions.				
4. Recorded the shade and type of artificial teeth in the patient's record.				
5. Prepared the case for shipment to the commercial laboratory.				
Try-In Visit(s)				
1. Before the patient's appointment, determined that the case had been returned from the laboratory.				
2. Assisted the dentist during try-in and adjustment of the appliance.				
3. When the appliance was removed, disinfected it and prepared the case to be returned to the laboratory for completion.				

Criteria	Peer	Self	Instructor	Comment
Delivery Visit				
1. Before the patient's appointment, determined that the completed case had been returned from the laboratory.				
2. Gathered the appropriate setup.				
3. Assisted in making any necessary adjustments.				
4. Provided the patient with home-care instructions.				

Total amount of points earned _____

Grade _____ *Instructor's initials* _____

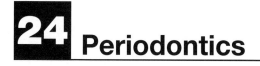

24 Periodontics

TRUE/FALSE

_____ 1. Kirkland knives are used during periodontal surgery.

_____ 2. Ultrasonic scalers increase operator hand fatigue.

_____ 3. Fluoride mouth rinses have been shown to reduce bleeding by delaying bacterial growth.

_____ 4. The scaling competency follows root planing.

_____ 5. A gingivoplasty involves the surgical reshaping and contouring of the gingival tissues.

FILL IN THE BLANK

6. _____ is an infection from the gingivae that progresses into the alveolar bone.

7. _____ is an inflammation of the gingiva.

8. _____ occur when the sulcus becomes deeper than normal.

9. A _____ is an instrument that is used to remove supragingival calculus.

10. _____ is the leading cause of tooth loss in adults.

11. A _____ curette is an instrument that is area specific and has one cutting edge.

12. A _____ is used to make bleeding points before a gingivectomy.

13. A _____ curette is an instrument with two cutting edges.

14. An _____ is an instrument that provides tactile information to the operator about the surface of the root.

15. An _____ knife is used to remove tissue from the interdental areas.

MULTIPLE CHOICE

16. Which of the following are reasons for periodontal surgery?
    a. reduce or eliminate pockets
    b. treat defects in the bone
    c. create new tissue attachment
    d. all of the above

17. Which of the following types of periodontal surgery removes bone?
    a. gingival graft
    b. laterally sliding flap
    c. osteoplasty
    d. ostectomy

18. Periodontal dressings are used to:
    a. hold the flaps in place
    b. protect the surgical site
    c. support mobile teeth during the healing process
    d. all of the above

19. Commonly used types of material for periodontal dressings are:
    a. zinc oxide and eugenol
    b. fluoride based
    c. non-eugenol
    d. a and c

20. The postoperative appointment after periodontal surgery is approximately:
    a. 24 hours
    b. 48 hours
    c. 1 week
    d. 1 month

Assisting With a Dental Prophylaxis

Performance Objective

The student will demonstrate the proper procedure for assisting with a dental prophylaxis.

Grading Criteria

3 Student meets most of the criteria without assistance.

2 Student requires assistance to meet the stated criteria.

1 Student did not prepare accordingly for the stated criteria.

0 Not applicable.

Criteria	Peer	Self	Instructor	Comment
1. Adjusted the light as necessary and was prepared to dry teeth with air when requested to do so.				
2. Provided retraction of the clips, tongue, and cheeks.				
3. Rinsed and evacuated fluid from the patient's mouth.				
4. Exchanged instruments with the operator.				
5. Passed the dental floss and/or tape.				
6. Reinforced oral hygiene instructions when requested to do so.				
7. Maintained patient comfort and followed appropriate infection-control measures throughout the procedure.				

Total amount of points earned _____

Grade _____ *Instructor's initials* _____

Assisting With Gingivectomy and Gingivoplasty

Performance Objective

The student will demonstrate the proper procedure for assisting with a gingivectomy and gingivoplasty.

Grading Criteria

3 Student meets most of the criteria without assistance.

2 Student requires assistance to meet the stated criteria.

1 Student did not prepare accordingly for the stated criteria.

0 Not applicable.

Criteria	Peer	Self	Instructor	Comment
1. Set out patient's health history, radiographs, and periodontal chart.				
2. Anticipated the operator's needs and was prepared to pass and retrieve surgical instruments.				
3. Had gauze ready to remove tissue from instruments.				
4. Provided oral evacuation and retraction.				
5. Irrigated with sterile saline.				
6. Assisted with suture placement.				
7. Placed, or assisted with placement of, the periodontal dressing.				
8. Provided postoperative instructions.				
9. Maintained patient comfort and followed appropriate infection-control measures throughout the procedure.				

Total amount of points earned _____

Grade _____ *Instructor's initials* _____

Preparing and Placing a Non-Eugenol Periodontal Dressing (Expanded Function)

Performance Objective

The student will demonstrate the proper procedure for preparing and placing a non-eugenol periodontal dressing.

Grading Criteria

3 Student meets most of the criteria without assistance.

2 Student requires assistance to meet the stated criteria.

1 Student did not prepare accordingly for the stated criteria.

0 Not applicable.

Criteria	Peer	Self	Instructor	Comment
Mixing				
1. Extruded equal lengths of the two pastes on a paper pad.				
2. Mixed the pastes until a uniform color was obtained (2 to 3 minutes).				
3. Placed the material in the paper cup.				
4. Lubricated gloved fingers with saline solution.				
5. Rolled the paste into strips.				
Placement				
1. Pressed small triangle-shaped pieces of dressing into the interproximal spaces.				
2. Adapted one end of the strip around the distal surface of the last tooth in the surgical site.				
3. Gently pressed the remainder of the strip along the incised gingival margin.				
4. Gently pressed the strip into the interproximal areas.				
5. Applied the second strip from the lingual surface.				
6. Joined the facial and lingual strips.				
7. Applied gentle pressure on the facial and lingual surfaces.				
8. Checked the dressing for overextension and interference.				
9. Removed any excess dressing and adjusted the new margins.				
10. Maintained patient comfort and followed appropriate infection-control measures throughout the procedure.				

Total amount of points earned _____

Grade _____ *Instructor's initials* _____

Removing a Periodontal Dressing

Performance Objective

The student will demonstrate the proper procedure for removing a periodontal dressing.

Grading Criteria

3 Student meets most of the criteria without assistance.

2 Student requires assistance to meet the stated criteria.

1 Student did not prepare accordingly for the stated criteria.

0 Not applicable.

Criteria	Peer	Self	Instructor	Comment
1. Gently inserted the spoon excavator under the margin.				
2. Used lateral pressure to gently pry the dressing away from the tissue.				
3. Checked for sutures and removed any present.				
4. Gently used dental floss to remove all fragments of dressing material.				
5. Irrigated the entire area gently with warm saline solution.				
6. Used the HVE tip or saliva ejector to remove fluid from the patient's mouth.				
7. Maintained patient comfort and followed appropriate infection-control measures throughout the procedure.				

Total amount of points earned _____

Grade _____ *Instructor's initials* _____

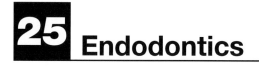

25 Endodontics

TRUE/FALSE

_____ 1. Endodontics is often referred to as root canal treatment.

_____ 2. A control tooth is used during each type of pulp testing procedure.

_____ 3. If decay is close to the pulp but has not penetrated it, the condition is termed irreversible pulpitis.

_____ 4. Necrosis is also referred to as nonvital.

_____ 5. Amalgam is used to obturate the pulpal canal.

_____ 6. Formocresol can be used as a sealer for a pulpotomy of permanent teeth.

_____ 7. A direct pulp cap is indicated when the pulp has been slightly exposed.

_____ 8. A pulpectomy is also referred to as root canal therapy.

_____ 9. If the tooth is nonvital, the endodontist may advise the patient to have inhalation sedation during the procedure.

_____ 10. The standard of care established by the ADA for endodontic treatment requires the use of a dental dam.

MATCHING

Match the following vitality tests with their descriptions.

_____ 11. Tapping on the tooth   A. Electric pulp test

_____ 12. Ice to the tooth   B. Palpation test

_____ 13. Small shock to the tooth   C. Heat test

         D. Percussion test

_____ 14. Firm pressure to the tooth   E. Cold test

_____ 15. High temperature to the tooth

Match the following instruments with their uses.

_____ 16. Hand instrument used to enter and locate canal openings   A. Endodontic spreader

         B. Broach

_____ 17. Paddle-shaped instrument for placement of temporary restorations   C. Endodontic explorer

         D. Glick #1

_____ 18. Hand instrument used to condense and adapt gutta-percha points to the canal   E. Endodontic plugger

_____ 19. Tiny fishhook barbs used to remove the bulk of the pulp tissue

_____ 20. Hand instrument used to obturate the canal by pressing the gutta-percha points in a lateral direction

21. The subjective portion of the examination includes evaluation of symptoms or problems described by the patient. List three specific questions to ask a patient.

22. Radiographs are exposed a minimum of four times at key points throughout an endodontic procedure. Name and describe each of the four radiographs.

Performance Objective

In states where it is legal, the student will demonstrate the proper procedure for performing an electric pulp vitality test.

Grading Criteria

3 Student meets most of the criteria without assistance.

2 Student requires assistance to meet the stated criteria.

1 Student did not prepare accordingly for the stated criteria.

0 Not applicable.

Criteria	Peer	Self	Instructor	Comment
1. Gathered the appropriate setup.				
2. Described the procedure to the patient.				
3. Identified the tooth to be tested and the appropriate control tooth.				
4. Isolated the teeth to be tested and dried them thoroughly.				
5. Set the control dial at zero.				
6. Placed a thin layer of toothpaste on the tip of the pulp tester electrode.				
7. Tested the control tooth first. Placed the tip of the electrode on the facial surface of the tooth at the cervical third.				
8. Gradually increased the level of the current until the patient felt a response. Recorded the response in the patient's record.				
9. Repeated the procedure on the suspected tooth and recorded the response on the patient's record.				
10. Maintained patient comfort and followed appropriate infection-control measures throughout the procedure.				

Total amount of points earned _____

Grade _____ *Instructor's initials* _____

Assisting in Root Canal Therapy

Performance Objective

The student will demonstrate the proper procedure for making pretreatment preparations and assisting in root canal therapy.

Grading Criteria

3 Student meets most of the criteria without assistance.

2 Student requires assistance to meet the stated criteria.

1 Student did not prepare accordingly for the stated criteria.

0 Not applicable.

Criteria	Peer	Self	Instructor	Comment
1. Prepared the appropriate setup.				
2. Assisted with the administration of a local anesthesia and the placing and disinfecting of the dental dam.				
3. Anticipated the dentist's needs.				
4. Maintained moisture control and a clear operating field throughout the procedure.				
5. Exchanged instruments as necessary.				
6. On request, irrigated the canals gently with a solution of sodium hypochlorite and used the HVE tip to remove the excess solution.				
7. On request, placed a rubber stop at the desired working length for that canal.				
8. Assisted in preparation of the trial-point radiograph.				
9. Exposed and processed the trial-point radiograph.				
10. At a signal from the endodontist, prepared the endodontic sealer.				
11. Dipped a file or Lentulo spiral into the cement and transferred it to the endodontist.				
12. Dipped the tip of the gutta-percha point into the sealer and transferred it to the endodontist.				
13. Transferred hand instruments and additional gutta-percha points to the endodontist.				
14. Continued the instrument exchange until the procedure was complete and the tooth was sealed with temporary cement.				
15. Exposed and processed a posttreatment radiograph.				
16. Gave the patient posttreatment instructions.				
17. Maintained patient comfort and followed appropriate infection-control measures throughout the procedure.				

Total amount of points earned _____

Grade _____ *Instructor's initials* _____

26 Oral and Maxillofacial Surgery

TRUE/FALSE

_____ 1. Oral surgical procedures should only take place in an operating room within a hospital setting.

_____ 2. All surgical instruments are classified as critical instruments and must be disinfected after each use.

_____ 3. Luxate means to rock back and forth.

_____ 4. Contact with anything that is not sterile will break the chain of asepsis and contaminate the surgical area.

_____ 5. A forceps extraction is performed on a tooth that is fully impacted.

_____ 6. Alveoloplasty is the procedure of surgically contouring and smoothing the remaining bone to provide a properly contoured ridge for the placement of a bridge, partial, or denture.

_____ 7. As a rule, if a scalpel has been used to cut tissue, then sutures are placed for proper healing.

_____ 8. Failure of a blood clot from an extraction can result in alveolitis.

_____ 9. Following a surgical procedure, home-care instructions should be provided over the telephone once the patient has arrived home.

_____ 10. Nonabsorbable suture materials include plain catgut, chromic catgut, and polydioxanone.

MATCHING

Match each surgical instrument to its use.

_____ 11. Trims alveolar bone

_____ 12. Removes root tips or fragments

_____ 13. Separates periosteum from bone

_____ 14. Grasps and holds items

_____ 15. Surgical knife

A. Periosteal elevator

B. Scalpel

C. Rongeur

D. Root tip picks

E. Hemostat

Match the surgical situation with its definition.

_____ 16. Dry socket

_____ 17. Covered by tissue or bone

_____ 18. Aseptic principle

_____ 19. Examination of tissue

_____ 20. Recontouring tissue and bone

A. Alveolitis

B. Biopsy

C. Alveoloplasty

D. Impaction

E. Sterile technique

SHORT ANSWER

21. List the instructions that should be given to a patient in regard to the control of bleeding.

22. List the instructions that should be given to a patient in regard to the control of swelling.

23. List the probable causes of alveolitis.

275

Performing a Surgical Scrub

Performance Objective

The student will demonstrate the proper procedure for performing a surgical scrub for a sterile surgical procedure.

Grading Criteria

3 Student meets most of the criteria without assistance.

2 Student requires assistance to meet the stated criteria.

1 Student did not prepare accordingly for the stated criteria.

0 Not applicable.

Criteria	Peer	Self	Instructor	Comment
1. Wet hands and forearms with warm water.				
2. Placed antimicrobial soap into hands.				
3. Used a surgical scrub brush to scrub hands and forearms for 8 minutes.				
4. Rinsed hands and forearms thoroughly with warm water, allowing the water to flow away from the hands.				
5. Accomplished additional washing in 3 minutes without a brush.				
6. Dried hands using a sterile, disposable towel.				

Total amount of points earned _____

Grade _____ *Instructor's initials* _____

Performing Sterile Gloving

Performance Objective

The student will demonstrate the proper procedure for gloving using a sterile technique.

Grading Criteria

3 Student meets most of the criteria without assistance.

2 Student requires assistance to meet the stated criteria.

1 Student did not prepare accordingly for the stated criteria.

0 Not applicable.

Criteria	Peer	Self	Instructor	Comment
1. Opened the glove package before the surgical scrub.				
2. Touched only the inside of the package after the surgical scrub.				
3. Gloved the dominant hand first, touching only the folded cuff.				
4. Placed the other glove on, touching only the sterile portion of the glove with the dominant hand.				
5. Unrolled the cuff from the gloves.				

Total amount of points earned _____

Grade _____ *Instructor's initials* _____

Assisting in a Surgical Extraction

Performance Objective

Provided with information concerning the type of surgery, the tooth, and the anesthetics used, the student will prepare the setup, prepare the patient, and assist in a surgical procedure.

Grading Criteria

3 Student meets most of the criteria without assistance.

2 Student requires assistance to meet the stated criteria.

1 Student did not prepare accordingly for the stated criteria.

0 Not applicable.

Criteria	Peer	Self	Instructor	Comment
Preparing the Treatment Room				
1. Prepared the treatment room.				
2. Kept instruments in their sterile wraps until ready for use. If a surgical tray was preset, opened the tray and placed a sterile towel over the instruments.				
3. Placed the appropriate local anesthetic on the tray.				
4. Placed the appropriate forceps on the tray.				
Preparing the Patient				
1. Seated the patient and placed a sterile patient drape or towel.				
2. Took the patient's vital signs and recorded them in the patient's record.				
3. Adjusted the dental chair to the proper position.				
4. Stayed with the patient until the dentist entered the treatment room.				
During the Surgical Procedure				
1. Maintained the chain of asepsis.				
2. Monitored vital signs.				
3. Aspirated and retracted as needed.				
4. Transferred and received instruments as needed.				
5. Assisted in suture placement as needed.				
6. Maintained a clear operating field with adequate light and irrigation.				

Criteria	Peer	Self	Instructor	Comment
7. Steadied the patient's head and mandible if necessary.				
8. Observed the patient's condition and anticipated the dentist's needs.				
9. Maintained patient comfort and followed appropriate infection-control measures throughout the procedure.				

Total amount of points earned _____

Grade _____ *Instructor's initials* _____

Assisting in Suture Placement

Performance Objective

The student will demonstrate the proper procedure for assisting the surgeon in suture placement.

Grading Criteria

3 Student meets most of the criteria without assistance.

2 Student requires assistance to meet the stated criteria.

1 Student did not prepare accordingly for the stated criteria.

0 Not applicable.

Criteria	Peer	Self	Instructor	Comment
1. Removed the suture material from the sterile package.				
2. Clamped the suture needle at the upper third.				
3. Transferred the needle holder to the surgeon.				
4. Retracted during suture placement.				
5. Cut suture where indicated by the surgeon.				
6. Placed suture material on tray.				
7. Recorded the number and types of sutures placed in the patient's record.				

Total amount of points earned _____

Grade _____ *Instructor's initials* _____

Performing Suture Removal (Expanded Function)

Performance Objective

The student will demonstrate the proper procedure for removing sutures.

Grading Criteria

3 Student meets most of the criteria without assistance.

2 Student requires assistance to meet the stated criteria.

1 Student did not prepare accordingly for the stated criteria.

0 Not applicable.

Criteria	Peer	Self	Instructor	Comment
1. Dentist examined the surgical site and instructed the assistant to remove the sutures.				
2. Wiped the area with an antiseptic agent.				
3. Held the suture away from the tissue with cotton pliers.				
4. Cut the suture with suture scissors, ensuring that the scissors were laying flat near the tissue.				
5. Grasped the knot with cotton pliers and removed it, keeping it away from the tissue.				
6. Counted the number of sutures removed and recorded it in the patient's record.				
7. Maintained patient comfort and followed appropriate infection-control measures throughout the procedure.				

Total amount of points earned _____

Grade _____ *Instructor's initials* _____

27 Pediatric Dentistry

TRUE/FALSE

_____ 1. Pediatric dentistry is the specialized area of dentistry limited to the care of children from infancy through adulthood.

_____ 2. Many pediatric dental offices are designed with several dental chairs arranged in one large treatment area or bay.

_____ 3. The pediatric dentist should refer patients with special needs to a specialist who has the background in working with these patients.

_____ 4. The child's parent or legal guardian must give his or her consent before any dental treatment can be provided for any child under the age of 14 years.

_____ 5. Behavioral assessment is used to evaluate the communication skills of the patient and determine whether behavior management techniques are necessary.

_____ 6. Prevention is one of the most encompassing areas for a pediatric dental practice.

_____ 7. Sealants are a common preventive procedure performed in a pediatric office.

_____ 8. The two matrix systems most commonly placed on primary teeth are the clear Mylar strip and Universal band.

_____ 9. Gold crowns are used in the treatment of badly decayed primary teeth.

_____ 10. Permanent teeth that have been avulsed have been knocked completely out of the mouth.

MATCHING

Match the following pediatric procedures with their description.

_____ 11. Fluoride treatment

_____ 12. Class II restoration

_____ 13. Pulpotomy

_____ 14. Space maintenance

_____ 15. Correcting a crossbite

A. Pulp therapy

B. Interceptive orthodontics

C. Preventive care

D. Restorative dentistry

E. Preventive orthodontics

SHORT ANSWER

16. List the stages of behavior.

17. Describe the techniques to be used when introducing a child to a radiographic procedure.

Assisting in the Pulpotomy of a Primary Tooth

Performance Objective

The student will demonstrate the proper technique when assisting in the pulpotomy of a primary tooth.

Grading Criteria

3 Student meets most of the criteria without assistance.

2 Student requires assistance to meet the stated criteria.

1 Student did not prepare accordingly for the stated criteria.

0 Not applicable.

Criteria	Peer	Self	Instructor	Comment
1. Gathered the appropriate setup.				
2. Assisted in the administration of the local anesthetic.				
3. Assisted in placement of or placed dental dam.				
4. Assisted in removal of dental caries.				
5. Used HVE and air-water syringe throughout procedure.				
6. Transferred instruments throughout the procedure.				
7. Prepared formocresol and cotton pellet and transferred when needed.				
8. Mixed ZOE for a base and transferred it to be placed.				
9. Maintained patient comfort and followed appropriate infection-control measures throughout the procedure.				

Total amount of points earned _____

Grade _____ *Instructor's initials* _____

Assisting in the Placement of a Stainless Steel Crown

Performance Objective

The student will demonstrate the proper technique when assisting in the preparation and placement of a stainless steel crown.

Grading Criteria

3 Student meets most of the criteria without assistance.

2 Student requires assistance to meet the stated criteria.

1 Student did not prepare accordingly for the stated criteria.

0 Not applicable.

Criteria	Peer	Self	Instructor	Comment
1. Gathered the appropriate setup.				
2. Assisted in the administration of the local anesthetic.				
3. Assisted in the sizing of the stainless steel crown.				
4. Transferred instruments as requested in the transfer zone.				
5. Assisted in trimming and contouring of the stainless steel crown.				
6. Prepared cement and assisted in the cementation of the stainless steel crown.				
7. Maintained patient comfort and followed appropriate infection-control measures throughout the procedure.				

Total amount of points earned _____

Grade _____ *Instructor's initials* _____

28 Orthodontics

TRUE/FALSE

_____ 1. Malocclusion is an abnormal or malpositioned relationship of the maxillary teeth to the mandibular teeth when occluded.

_____ 2. Motivation for seeking orthodontic treatment is not an important factor.

_____ 3. The purpose of the orthodontic clinical exam is to document and evaluate the facial aspects, the occlusal relationship, and the functional characteristics of the jaws.

_____ 4. There are four standard extraoral photographs taken during the clinical examination.

_____ 5. Fixed appliances are commonly known as braces.

_____ 6. The radiograph that is taken routinely in the orthodontic clinical exam is the panoramic.

_____ 7. Brackets are bonded directly to the lingual surface of anterior and premolar teeth.

_____ 8. A week before the banding appointment, a separator is placed to force the mesial and distal spaces of the tooth slightly apart.

_____ 9. During orthodontic treatment, specific foods to be avoided are mashed potatoes, fruit, and pasta.

_____ 10. Loose bands can result from a break in the cement seal or from poor eating habits.

MATCHING

Match each instrument with its use.

_____ 11. Aids in seating a molar band

_____ 12. Tucks the twisted ligature tie under the arch wire

_____ 13. Cuts the end of the arch wire

_____ 14. Used in placing the arch wire

_____ 15. Helps form and bend wires

A. Distal end cutter

B. Weingart pliers

C. Bite stick

D. Ligature director

E. Bird beak pliers

Match the fixed appliance with its description.

_____ 16. Holds the end of the arch wire and any additional power products

_____ 17. Holds the arch wire in place within the bracket

_____ 18. Creates tooth movement

_____ 19. Attachment for the arch wire

_____ 20. Creates space to seat bands

A. Bracket

B. Arch wire

C. Separator

D. Ligature tie

E. Molar band

SHORT ANSWER

21. What are the three major sources of information used to make a diagnosis?

22. At each adjustment appointment, it is the responsibility of the chairside assistant to check the patient's appliance. What specific things should the assistant look for?

Performance Objective

The student will demonstrate the proper technique when placing separators.

Grading Criteria

3 Student meets most of the criteria without assistance.

2 Student requires assistance to meet the stated criteria.

1 Student did not prepare accordingly for the stated criteria.

0 Not applicable.

Criteria	Peer	Self	Instructor	Comment
1. Gathered the appropriate setup.				
2. Explained the procedure to the patient.				
3. Carried the separator with the appropriate instrument for placement.				
4. Inserted the separator below the proximal contact.				
5. Recorded the amount of separators placed in the patient record.				
6. Provided postoperative instructions to the patient.				
7. Maintained patient comfort and followed appropriate infection-control measures throughout the procedure.				

Total amount of points earned _____

Grade _____ *Instructor's initials* _____

Performance Objective

The student will prepare the appropriate setup and assist in the cementation of orthodontic bands.

Grading Criteria

3 Student meets most of the criteria without assistance.

2 Student requires assistance to meet the stated criteria.

1 Student did not prepare accordingly for the stated criteria.

0 Not applicable.

Criteria	Peer	Self	Instructor	Comment
1. Gathered the appropriate setup.				
2. Placed each preselected orthodontic band on a small square of masking tape with the occlusal surface on the tape.				
3. Wiped any buccal tubes or attachments with lip balm.				
4. Mixed the cement according to the manufacturer's instructions.				
5. Loaded the bands with cement correctly by flowing cement into the band.				
6. Transferred the band correctly.				
7. For a maxillary band, transferred the band pusher.				
8. For a mandibular band, transferred the band seater.				
9. Repeated the process until all bands were cemented.				
10. Cleaned the cement spatula and slab.				
11. Used a scaler or explorer to remove the excess cement on the enamel surfaces, then rinsed the patient's mouth.				
12. Maintained patient comfort and followed appropriate infection-control measures throughout the procedure.				

Total amount of points earned _____

Grade _____ *Instructor's initials* _____

Assisting in the Direct Bonding of Orthodontic Brackets

Performance Objective

The student will prepare the appropriate setup and assist in the bonding of orthodontic brackets.

Grading Criteria

3 Student meets most of the criteria without assistance.

2 Student requires assistance to meet the stated criteria.

1 Student did not prepare accordingly for the stated criteria.

0 Not applicable.

Criteria	Peer	Self	Instructor	Comment
1. Gathered the appropriate setup.				
2. If stain or plaque was present, prepared the tooth surfaces using a rubber cup and a pumice slurry.				
3. Isolated the teeth.				
4. Assisted throughout the etching of the teeth.				
5. Applied a small quantity of bonding material on the back of the bracket.				
6. Used bracket placement tweezers to transfer the brackets to the orthodontist.				
7. Transferred an orthodontic scaler for final placement and the removal of excess bonding material.				
8. Maintained patient comfort and followed appropriate infection-control measures throughout the procedure.				

Total amount of points earned _____

Grade _____ *Instructor's initials* _____

Placing and Removing Ligature Wires (Expanded Function)

Performance Objective

The student will demonstrate the proper technique when placing and removing ligature wires.

Grading Criteria

3 Student meets most of the criteria without assistance.

2 Student requires assistance to meet the stated criteria.

1 Student did not prepare accordingly for the stated criteria.

0 Not applicable.

Criteria	Peer	Self	Instructor	Comment
Placing the Ligature Wires				
1. Gathered the appropriate setup.				
2. Placed the ligature wire around the bracket and used the ligature director to push the wire against the tie wing.				
3. Properly twisted the ends of the ligature together.				
4. Used the hemostat to twist the wire snugly against the bracket. Repeated the procedure until all brackets were ligated.				
5. Used a ligature cutter to cut the excess wire, leaving a 4- to 5-mm pigtail.				
6. Tucked the pigtails under the arch wire using the correct instruments.				
7. Determined that nothing was protruding that might injure the patient.				
Removing the Ligature Wire				
1. Held the ligature cutter properly and used the beaks of the pliers to cut the wire at the easiest access.				
2. Carefully unwrapped the ligature and removed it.				
3. Did not twist or pull as the ligatures were cut and removed.				
4. Continued cutting and removing until all brackets were untied.				
5. Maintained patient comfort and followed appropriate infection-control measures throughout the procedure.				

Total amount of points earned _____

Grade _____ *Instructor's initials* _____

29 The Job Search

TRUE / FALSE

_____ 1. Many dental assistants find personal pride and fulfillment by joining a private practice.

_____ 2. Dental insurance companies hire dental assistants with knowledge of the processing of claims and customer service.

_____ 3. Your first contact with a prospective employer will probably be by e-mail.

_____ 4. A cover letter serves to introduce you to your prospective employer.

_____ 5. A résumé communicates a minimum amount of information through a maximum number of words.

_____ 6. There is only one correct way to write a résumé.

_____ 7. Within your résumé, you should list your most recent to least recent work experiences.

_____ 8. CPR would be considered a certification that should be listed on your résumé.

_____ 9. Volunteer work would not be listed on your résumé because it does not pertain to dentistry.

_____ 10. You should plan to arrive 15 minutes before the scheduled time of an interview.

SHORT ANSWER

11. Name the various career opportunities that a dental assistant can pursue.

12. List the various sources that you can refer to for employment.

13. Give 10 tips for having a good interview.

Preparing a Professional Résumé

Performance Objective

Given a computer, printer, and paper, the student will prepare a one-page résumé.

Grading Criteria

3 Student meets most of the criteria without assistance.

2 Student requires assistance to meet the stated criteria.

1 Student did not prepare accordingly for the stated criteria.

0 Not applicable.

Criteria	Peer	Self	Instructor	Comment
1. Used common typefaces.				
2. Used a 10-, 12-, or 14-point font size.				
3. Used 1-inch margins on all sides.				
4. Résumé was one page in length.				
5. Résumé was neat and error free.				
6. Résumé was concise and easy to read.				

Total amount of points earned _____

Grade _____ Instructor's initials _____

Bones of the Skull

Describe the location of the following cranial bones:

1. Frontal
2. Temporal
3. Parietal
4. Sphenoid
5. Occipital
6. Ethmoid

Types of Teeth

Describe the location and function of the four types of teeth:

1. Incisors
2. Premolars
3. Canine
4. Molars

Bones of the Face

Describe the location of the following facial bones:

1. Zygomatic
2. Nasal
3. Inferior conchae
4. Maxillary
5. Lacrimal
6. Mandible
7. Palatine
8. Vomer

Surfaces of Teeth

Describe the surface location of the six types of teeth.

1. Facial
2. Lingual
3. Occlusal
4. Incisal
5. Mesial
6. Distal

Tissues of the Teeth

Identify the four tissues of the teeth and their makeup.

Tooth Eruption

Describe the age of eruption for the following permanent maxillary and mandibular teeth.

1. Central incisors
2. Canines
3. Second premolars
4. Second molars
5. Lateral incisors
6. First premolars
7. First molars
8. Third molars

Types of Teeth

1. Front of mouth/cutting food
2. Corner of mouth/cutting and tearing
3. Back of mouth/grasping and tearing
4. Back of mouth/chewing and grinding

Surfaces of Teeth

1. Toward the lips
2. Toward the tongue
3. Back chewing surface
4. Front chewing surface
5. Interproximal surface closest to midline
6. Interproximal surface away from midline

Tooth Eruption

1. 6–8 years
2. 9–12 years
3. 10–13 years
4. 11–13 years
5. 7–9 years
6. 10–11 years
7. 6–17 years
8. 17–21 years

Bones of the Skull

1. Forehead
2. Sides
3. Roof
4. Anterior base
5. Base
6. Orbit and floor

Bones of the Face

1. Cheeks
2. Nose
3. Interior nose
4. Upper jaw
5. Orbit
6. Lower jaw
7. Hard palate
8. Base of nose

Tissues of the Teeth

1. Enamel—the outer covering of the coronal portion of the tooth
2. Dentin—makes up most of the tooth and is reparative
3. Cementum—the outer layer of the root structure for attachment
4. Pulp—contains the nerves and blood of the tooth

Emergency Preparedness

Describe the roles of each professional in an emergency situation.

1. Business assistant

2. Chairside assistant

3. Dentist

Emergency Situation

How would you respond to a patient with hypoglycemia?

Cardiopulmonary Resuscitation

Describe the *ABCDs* of CPR.

Emergency Situation

How would you respond to a patient with syncope?

Emergency Drugs

The following drugs can be found in an emergency kit. For what emergency is each drug prepared?

1. Epinephrine

2. Antihistamine

3. Diazepam

4. Nitroglycerin

5. Inhaler

6. Ammonia inhalant

Emergency Situation

How would you respond to a patient with anaphylaxis?

Emergency Situation

1. Administer concentrated sugar under patient's tongue.
2. Ready CPR if needed.
3. Monitor and record vital signs.

Cardiopulmonary Resuscitation

A = Airway. Check to make sure patient's airway is open.

B = Breathing. Identify if patient is breathing on his or her own. If not, respond by giving two breaths.

C = Circulation. Identify a pulse. If no pulse, respond by administering chest compressions.

D = Defibrillation. Administer external defibrillation, if necessary.

Emergency Drugs

1. Acute allergic reaction
2. Allergic response
3. Seizure
4. Chest pain
5. Asthma attack
6. Respiratory stimulant

Emergency Preparedness

1. Calls emergency services.
2. Retrieves oxygen/drug kit and assesses patient.
3. Remains with patient and determines patient needs.

Emergency Situation

1. Place patient in supine position.
2. Prepare ammonia inhalant.
3. Prepare oxygen if needed.
4. Monitor and record vital signs.

Emergency Situation

1. Position patient in supine position.
2. Prepare epinephrine for administration.
3. Prepare for CPR if needed.
4. Monitor and record vital signs.

Disease Transmission

Describe the following methods of disease transmission.

1. Direct
2. Indirect
3. Splash/splatter
4. Airborne
5. Dental unit waterlines

Diseases of Major Concern

Describe the following diseases and their effects.

1. Hepatitis B
2. Human immunodeficiency virus
3. Tuberculosis

Disinfection Procedures

1. Define disinfection.
2. Describe the spray-wipe-spray technique.

Sterilization Procedures

Describe the following sterilization methods:

1. Steam sterilization
2. Chemical vapor sterilization
3. Dry-heat sterilization

Hazard Communication

Describe the following parts of a hazard communication program.

1. Written program
2. Chemical inventory
3. MSDS
4. Labeling
5. Training

Personal Protective Equipment

What are the four components of PPE, and how do they protect the caregiver?

Disinfection Procedures

1. Killing or inhibiting pathogens from growth by the use of a chemical agent
2. Spray—Thoroughly spray the surface.
   Wipe—Wipe the surface clean.
   Spray—Spray with disinfectant for recommended time.

Sterilization Procedures

1. Superheated steam under pressure for a recommended time (250° F, 20 minutes, 15–20 PSI)
2. Superheated chemical under pressure for a recommended time (270° F, 20–40 minutes, 20 PSI)
3. Superheat with no moisture or chemical for a recommended time (340° F, 60 minutes)

Hazard Communication

1. Document maintained to identify employees who are exposed to hazardous materials
2. Comprehensive list of chemicals used in the dental office
3. Information by the manufacturer describing the physical and chemical properties of a product
4. All containers labeled with name of product and any hazardous material
5. Training required for (1) new employees, (2) when a new chemical is acquired, and (3) yearly for continuing education

Disease Transmission

1. Contact with infectious lesions
2. Contact with a contaminated object
3. Blood, saliva, and body fluids
4. Microorganisms in sprays, mists, and aerosols
5. Microorganisms in water from dental unit

Diseases of Major Concern

1. Bloodborne virus that affects the liver and is transmitted by body fluids
2. Bloodborne virus that affects the immune system and is transmitted by body fluids
3. Bacterial infection that mostly affects the lungs

Personal Protective Equipment

1. Protective clothing protects the skin and underclothing from exposure.
2. A protective mask prevents the inhalation of infectious organisms.
3. Protective eyewear protects the eye from aerosol and debris.
4. Protective gloves prevent direct contact with contaminated objects.

Radiation Protection

1. Define three types of radiation protection methods for the patient.

2. Define two types of radiation protection methods for the operator.

Concept of Paralleling Technique

Describe the positioning of the film, tooth, and central ray for the paralleling technique.

Concept of Bisecting Technique

Describe the positioning of the film, tooth, and central ray for the bisecting technique.

Processing Radiographs

1. Describe the role of developer in the processing of exposed radiographs.

2. Describe the role of fixer in the processing of exposed radiographs.

Technique Errors

Describe how the following errors occur:

1. Elongation   5. Foreshortening

2. Overlapping   6. Herringbone pattern

3. Underexposure   7. Double exposure

4. Cone cutting   8. Bent film

Types of Extraoral Films

Define the use for the following extraoral films:

1. Panoramic   2. Cephalometric   3. Tomogram

Processing Radiographs

1. Developer reacts with silver halide crystals on the film that were affected by radiation. These crystals form the images.
2. Fixer removes any crystals that did not react, hardens the emulsion, and preserves the image.

Radiation Protection

1.
   - Proper film-exposure technique
   - Use of film-holding instruments
   - Lead apron and thyroid collar

2.
   - Personnel monitoring
   - Equipment monitoring

Technique Errors

1. Not enough vertical angulation
2. Central ray not directed through interproximal space
3. Settings too low
4. X-ray beam did not expose entire film
5. Too much vertical angulation
6. Film reversed
7. Film exposed twice
8. Film bent in mouth

Concept of Paralleling Technique

- The film is parallel to the long axis of the tooth.
- The x-ray beam is directed to the right angle of the film and the long axis of the tooth.

Types of Extraoral Films

1. Provides a view of the entire maxilla and mandible
2. Provides a lateral view of the skull
3. Provides a view of sections of the temporomandibular joint (TMJ)

Concept of Bisecting Technique

- The film is angled to the long axis of the tooth.
- The space between the film and tooth is bisected.
- The x-ray beam is directed perpendicular to the bisecting line.

Hand Cutting Instruments

Define the use for the following instruments:

1. Excavator
2. Hatchet
3. Hoe
4. Chisel
5. Gingival margin trimmer

Endodontic Instruments

Identify the use for the following instruments:

1. Broach
2. File
3. Rubber stopper
4. Endodontic explorer
5. Spreader
6. Plugger

Restorative Instruments

Define the use for the following instruments:

1. Amalgam carrier
2. Amalgam condenser
3. Burnisher
4. Discoid-cleoid carver
5. Hollenback carver
6. Composite instrument

Oral Surgery Instruments

Identify the use for the following instruments:

1. Elevator
2. Forceps
3. Surgical curette
4. Rongeur
5. Bone file
6. Scalpel
7. Hemostat
8. Needle holder

Handpiece and Rotary Instruments

Define the use for the following instruments:

1. High-speed handpiece
2. Low-speed handpiece
3. Straight attachment
4. Contra-angle attachment
5. Friction-grip bur
6. Latch-type bur

Orthodontic Instruments

Identify the use for the following instruments:

1. Ligature director
2. Band plugger
3. Bite stick
4. Bird beak pliers
5. Distal end cutter
6. Pin and ligature cutter
7. Band remover
8. Howe pliers

Endodontic Instruments

1. To remove most of pulp tissue
2. To smooth and enlarge the canal
3. Small piece of rubber to measure the length of the file
4. Long and straight explorer to locate canal openings
5. Pointed end to assist in filling the canal
6. Flat end to assist in filling the canal

Oral Surgery Instruments

1. To reflect and retract the periosteum from the bone
2. To remove the tooth from the socket
3. To clean and remove diseased tissue from the socket
4. To trim alveolar bone
5. To smooth the surface of the bone
6. Surgical knife
7. To grasp and hold items
8. To hold the surgical needle firmly during suturing

Orthodontic Instruments

1. To guide and tuck ligature ties under the archwire
2. To aid in seating molar bands
3. To aid in seating molar bands
4. To form and bend the archwire
5. To cut and hold the end of the archwire
6. To cut ligature wire
7. To remove bands
8. Versatile pliers used to bend wires

Hand Cutting Instruments

1. To remove decay and debris from the tooth
2. To smooth the walls and floors of a prepared tooth
3. To smooth the floors of a prepared tooth
4. To smooth the enamel margin, and form sharp lines, point angles, and retention grooves
5. To place bevels along the gingival margin

Restorative Instruments

1. To carry amalgam to the prepared tooth
2. To pack amalgam into the tooth
3. To smooth amalgam
4. To carve the occlusal anatomy of amalgam
5. To carve the interproximal anatomy of amalgam
6. To place composite material into the prepared tooth

Handpiece and Rotary Instruments

1. Runs at 450,000 rpm to remove decay and large amount of tooth structure
2. Runs at 25,000 rpm to finish, contour, and polish
3. Fits on low-speed handpiece, and holds long-shank lab burs
4. Fits on low-speed handpiece, and holds latch-type burs, prophy cups, and brushes
5. Available in assorted shapes and fits on high-speed handpiece
6. Available in assorted shapes and fits on contra-angle of low-speed handpiece

Preventive Materials

Describe the following preventive materials and their use:

1. Systemic fluoride
2. Topical fluoride
3. Sealants

Amalgam

Describe the makeup of amalgam.

Impression Materials

Describe the following impression materials and their use:

1. Hydrocolloids
2. Reversible hydrocolloids
3. Elastomeric

Composite Resin

Describe the makeup of composite resin.

Laboratory Procedures

Describe the following procedures completed in the dental laboratory:

1. Diagnostic cast
2. Custom tray
3. Temporary crown
4. Vacuum-formed tray

Cements

Identify the use for the following cements:

1. Glass ionomer
2. Zinc phosphate
3. Zinc-oxide eugenol
4. Polycarboxylate
5. Intermediate restorative material

Preventive Materials

1. Mineral found in water, food, and supplements to prevent decay

2. Mineral found in toothpaste, mouthrinses, concentrated gel, and foam to prevent decay

3. Liquid resin applied and cured in the pits and fissures of teeth to prevent decay

Impression Materials

1. Referred to as alginate; used to obtain preliminary impressions for diagnostic purposes

2. Type of impression material with the ability to change its physical state

3. Referred to as a final impression; these materials get the most accurate impression

Laboratory Procedures

1. To diagnose, to fabricate an appliance, and for records

2. Type of tray that is fabricated specifically for a patient's mouth

3. Temporary coverage of a tooth or teeth made from acrylic or prefabricated material

4. Light-gauge plastic material that is form-fitted over a cast and then trimmed to fit over a patient arch

Amalgam

- Silver (to strengthen)
- Tin (to strengthen, and for workability)
- Copper (to strengthen, and for low corrosive properties)
- Mercury (to provide easy application and adaptability to tooth structure)

Composite Resin

- Resin matrix (also known as BIS-GMA, a material used to make synthetic resins)
- Inorganic fillers (quartz, glass, silica)
- Coupling agent (to strengthen and chemically bond the filler to the resin matrix)

Cements

1. Permanent cementation, restorations, liners, and bonding

2. Permanent cementation and insulating base

3. Permanent cementation, temporary cementation, and insulating base

4. Permanent cementation and insulating base

5. Temporary restorative material

Preventive Procedures

Define the following procedures:

1. Flossing
2. Toothbrushing
3. Coronal polishing
4. Fluoride treatment

Oral Surgery

Define the following procedures:

1. Forceps extraction
2. Impaction
3. Alveoloplasty
4. Suture
5. Biopsy

Restorative Classifications

Define the following cavity classifications:

1. Class I restorations
2. Class II restorations
3. Class III restorations
4. Class IV restorations
5. Class V restorations
6. Class VI restorations

Endodontics

Define the following procedures:

1. Indirect pulp capping
2. Direct pulp capping
3. Pulpotomy
4. Pulpectomy
5. Apicoectomy

Prosthodontics

Define the following procedures:

1. Inlay
2. Onlay
3. Veneer
4. Crown
5. Fixed bridge
6. Partial denture
7. Full denture

Periodontics

Define the following procedures:

1. Scaling
2. Root planing
3. Gingival curettage
4. Gingivectomy
5. Gingivoplasty
6. Osteoplasty

Oral Surgery

1. Removal of a fully erupted tooth

2. Removal of a tooth partially or totally covered by tissue and bone

3. Surgical contour of the bone and soft tissue after an extraction

4. Application of a material to control bleeding and promote healing

5. Surgical removal of tissue for analysis

Endodontics

1. Application of calcium hydroxide when the dental pulp is not exposed

2. Application of calcium hydroxide when the dental pulp has a slight exposure

3. Partial removal of the dental pulp

4. Complete removal of the dental pulp

5. Surgical removal of the apical portion of the root

Periodontics

1. Removal of calculus from a tooth surface

2. Removal of calculus and necrotic cementum

3. Removal of necrotic tissue from the gingival wall of the periodontal pocket

4. Surgical removal of diseased gingiva

5. Surgical reshaping of the gingival tissues

6. Surgical reshaping of bone

Preventive Procedures

1. To remove plaque from interproximal tooth surfaces

2. To remove plaque from tooth surfaces

3. To remove plaque and stains from teeth after calculus is removed

4. To apply topical fluoride to clean teeth

Restorative Classifications

1. Pit-and-fissure cavities

2. Posterior interproximal cavities

3. Anterior interproximal cavities

4. Anterior interproximal cavities involving the incisal edge

5. Smooth-surface cavities

6. Cavities or abrasions involving the incisal edge or occlusal cusp

Prosthodontics

1. Fixed restoration involving a portion of the occlusal and interproximal surface

2. Fixed restoration involving most of the occlusal and interproximal surface

3. Thin-shelled, tooth-colored restoration for facial surfaces

4. Fixed restoration covering all of the anatomic crown of a tooth

5. Fixed restoration replacing one or more teeth in the same arch

6. Removable prosthesis replacing one or more teeth in the same arch

7. Removable prosthesis replacing all teeth in the same arch